FITNESS COMPETITIONS *NATURALLY*

Dr. Katelyn Butler-Birmingham, ND

CreateSpace

Dr. Katelyn Butler-Birmingham

ISBN: 978-1-7753220-1-7

Editor: Linda M. Verde, CopyWriteEdit

Photo Credits:
    Front Cover and The Wrap Up section:
        Cameron Shaver from Kitchener Muscle
    Back Cover: Paula Tizzard Photography

    Published by Katelyn Butler-Birmingham at
        CreateSpace
        May 2018

This book is dedicated to you, the Reader!

Dr. Katelyn Butler-Birmingham

Thank you . . .

to my Mom who taught me to do what I feel is right,
even if I'm standing alone; to my Dad for passing on
his incredible determination; to my Love, Patrick,
for his support and humour throughout this
journey; and, to my friends, family and co-workers
for listening to me yammer on about this and
sharing in my excitement! Thanks to Sheila, for
being my amazing and patient test reader.

Special thanks to Karen Alexander, a coach and a
friend – I could not have done it without you!

Table of Contents

Introduction

I'm writing this book as a guide for people who are interested in **fitness competitions**, who want to know what it is like to train and compete, and how it can be **done all naturally**. Just because something has always been done, doesn't make it the right thing for you. Being a Naturopath, I've gotten used to being outside the box, and I encourage you to join me! See what kind of transformation your body can make using just food, water and even a little salt.

If you are new to the fitness competition world, you probably have a lot of questions. I was lucky enough to have people around me who have done shows, but if you are starting out, this book will answer many of your questions and get you headed down the right path.

I debated for a time about the format for this book. I wasn't sure if it was going to be completely practical or not. I settled on a mix of practical guide and personal experience so you get a real sense of the dos and don'ts of natural fitness competing. The personal experience is in the form of diary entries (in italics).

I haven't kept a diary for many years – pretty much since elementary school, where I'd write about my crushes – but for some reason I decided to keep one for this experience. Danielle, one of the chiropractic health assistants at Martin Wellness bought us all inspirational notebooks for Christmas 2016; mine said "Be so good they can't ignore you." That became my journal and my theme for 2017.

Included are some of my own personal notes and feelings experienced along this journey, interspersed with practical information that you need to know – from doing your first show, to self-care and recovery. While writing my diary I had no idea I would be publishing any of it, but I have left my experiences expressed in the entries uncensored!

My Story

As a child I was adventurous and active – always running around and playing sports with the boys at recess. I got into soccer when I was about eight, then in high school I played soccer, basketball and volleyball. In Grade 11, my good friend, Aurelie, introduced me to Pilates. I had never heard of it, but we started doing it together in the computer labs after school. This was my introduction to 'working out'; everything before that was organized sports. She also got me free day-passes to her gym and so began my journey in the fitness world.

Pilates and working out provided a new challenge. I was eager to see how it improved my athletic ability. In university, the sports dwindled to soccer only, but I took Kinesiology Pre-Health Co-op at the University of Waterloo to explore my love of sport and science combined. While there, I got my personal training certificate in 2008 and dabbled in training others, but mostly used it to fine-tune my own workouts.

Continuing my education, I went on to study Naturopathic Medicine at the Canadian College of Naturopathic Medicine. During my last year, I focused in Sports Medicine. After graduation, I started my practice in November 2015 and love working with athletes and people who are looking to live a healthy lifestyle, but need help getting started. To complement my practice, I started offering personal training part-time at Wellington Fitness in London, Ontario.

Now let's jump forward to January 2015 – the time of year for New Year's resolutions. I've never been much for them, but that particular year I told myself that within two years I wanted to look like the women in *Na Na*, the Trey Songz video. In this video, the women look amazing and are incredibly fit! Well, 2015 came and went; then 2016 almost came and went, but luckily I work with Karen and Saadiya. These two personal trainers, who had done a fitness competition show a few years earlier, offered to help me. That started a new chapter in my life, *natural fitness competitions*; first the Stephanie Worsfold Classic and later the KW Oktoberfest.

I've always been a practise-what-you-preach type of person and expect that from others. If I didn't believe and live the message I was promoting, I wouldn't feel comfortable treating patients, personal training, or teaching canfitpro's™ course for Healthy Eating and Weight Loss Coach. To me, the best way to help people is to understand where they're coming from, see their potential, and let them learn from your example – whether that means your own personal mistakes or your triumphs.

Like my sister, you might wonder why I'd want to enter a fitness competition. One day she asked me, "Why the heck would you want to do this? You're standing up there in a bikini, being judged. I could never do that." Hmm. Well, good question.

Why did I want to participate in a show? If you are reading this book, you probably have your own reasons why. For me, initially I only saw the challenge of getting more fit, and doing it all naturally. It had always been something I thought was out of reach, but now I had help and encouragement. Being on-stage in a bikini wasn't even a consideration at that point. When my bikini arrived in the mail, that's when it hit me. I'd be on-stage in this tiny, tiny, TINY suit! Surprisingly, once you have experienced the spray tan, wearing the bikini feels like A LOT of clothes. You'll see what I mean later.

PART I: First Show Everrr!

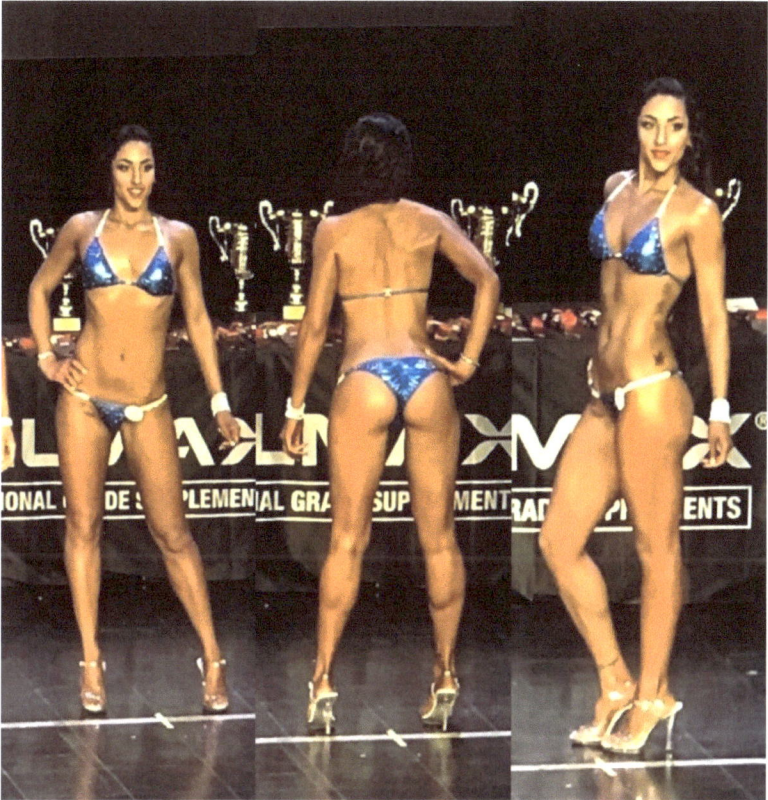

Stephanie Worsfold Natural Classic May 2017

"As with any new challenge, be prepared for a
physical, mental and emotional ride!"
– Dr. Katelyn Butler-Birmingham, ND

What You Need to Know

Before you jump right into the competition world, make sure to do your research. Gather the information you need and prepare yourself for a mental, emotional and physical ride. Once you get started, you learn a lot about yourself and the people surrounding you. Sometimes, how you think, how you look and how you feel is a roller coaster ride, but it's up to you to ensure that you take away as much as you can from the ups and downs. Also, you may not react the same way in a second show as you do in your first show.

As I started writing this book, I was preparing for my second show and already I felt different; more confident and ready than I felt the first time. This time, I knew what to expect from my body. I had a pretty good idea of where my mind goes, and yes it goes to a hungry, grumpy and tired place near the end, but I was eager to better myself for the next competition. There are many surprises along your journey. Here, at least, I can help you mitigate a few.

> *Gather the information you need and prepare yourself for a mental, emotional and physical ride.*

Cost

I was very fortunate to have Karen and Saadiya who helped me with posing, diet and workouts. This saved me a bundle of money, but if you are venturing out on your own, here are some costs to include in your budget.

Personal Trainer – If you are the kind of person who needs a personal trainer to stay on track, expect to pay anywhere from $1,300-6,000 depending on how long it takes you to prepare. Preparation time depends on the weight loss required. I definitely recommend taking your time. Rushing in the last moments to lose weight is stressful.

Coach – This is the person who helps you with diet and workouts, some coaches even teach posing. They develop plans for you, and you carry out the plans on the front lines. Coaches have different fees. Some require a lump sum payment of $300-500, others accept monthly payments of $120-150. They also may charge you $90-100 to have them backstage at the show. Note: Even if you're a personal trainer yourself, I still recommend having someone else do your workout plan for you. Why? Because they'll be able to take your measurements, make changes to your routine based on how you look, and come up with creative plans when you're stuck.

Posing class – You can literally win or lose on posing. Even with the best physique in the group, if your posing is off – it's game over. Many coaches that live out of town do distance training and keep up with you via Skype and pictures. If you need extra help with posing, definitely take a class or individual lessons. I found a group class in Kitchener taught by

Melissa Shadd for $20. Individual classes range from $45-60 per hour. Once you have the posing basics down, practise, Practise, PRACTISE! Use a mirror at first, then take it away and feel what your body needs to do. The footwork and hand positions need to be second nature to you. I practised every other day for a month leading up to the show. But take as much time as you need to feel comfortable in the heels that are required (see Clear heels below).

Gym membership – it is possible to get the results you want with a very well equipped home gym, but most people need a gym membership to have access to the variety of machines and weights needed. Gym membership prices vary from $11-60 per month.

Supplements/ergogenic aids – I used professional grade fish oil and magnesium by NFH, Vitamin C, Kaizen whey protein and Karbolyn for the first competition. This cost $50 per month on average. The least expensive place to get Kaizen is Costco.

Keep in mind, what worked for me won't necessarily be safe and/or effective for you. Always consult a healthcare professional when considering taking any new supplements or exercise aids. You never know what products may interact with any current medications you are taking, or may just be a waste of money for you – each product is different and how it reacts in the body is specific to the individual. For example, not everyone responds to supplements or absorbs them at the same rate. Your current health, past medical history, experience working out, age and sex are important factors to consider.

Food scale – the most cost effective one I found was from Walmart at $20. It is tempting to just 'eyeball' your portions or use hand measurements, but when it comes down to the crunch, every gram and ounce counts. So measure and be accurate.

Bikini/Figure suit – The huge price range for these goes from $110-3,000 or more. The range is so vast because you can get one-of-a-kind suits, tailored perfectly for you with jewels and sparkles galore. I didn't want to spend a fortune on my suits, so I bought them online from Etsy (Etsy.com). Search "fitness competition suits" and many choices come up. Make sure you have your measurements ready, and specify half-coverage for the bikini bottoms.

I got both of my suits from Flexfit Bikinis – one of them took two weeks to arrive ($109.53) and was perfect, the other ($96.17) took one month and arrived damaged. Luckily they offered to send new connectors, but that meant an additional waiting time of two weeks. If you decide to purchase online, be prepared for this and buy early! I had the suits modified and reinforced by Christy Wolfe in Dutton, Ontario, for $20. If you need alterations to make your suit fit just right, and want quick, professional service, contact her at wolfdsigns@hotmail.com. Many things can happen on-stage; flashing the public would probably be one of the worst. So, make sure your suit is secure, even if it means reinforcing it again yourself.

Clear heels – The shoes have to be clear so they don't distract from your body. The heels must be at least five inches high. I suggest buying a pair with an ankle strap – although there may be other times you want to channel Cinderella, I doubt losing a shoe on-stage is one of them. I looked at buying shoes online, but had such good customer service at London's Glamour and Fashion that I bought them there for $76.84. Prices online varied from $60-120.

Self-care – If you don't have benefits, plan for extended healthcare visits like chiropractic, massage and naturopathic. Costs vary on services used, but with a combination of the above, I spent probably $250-350 per month as I got closer to the show.

Competition spray tan – Ensure the tanning place you choose specializes in this type of tan. It is much darker than a regular spray tan and they spray it in a way to highlight your physique. I paid $89.99 plus tax at Hollywood Tan with $25 for a next-day touch-up, if needed.

With my skin colour, I still needed a spray tan. The lights really wash you out and the spray helps mask any tan lines you may have that take away from the look of your muscle definition. I didn't have my face sprayed, but for lighter skin I suggest a light spray on the face. For the second show I had my spray tan done at Shoreline Glow in Kitchener, Ontario. She had a promotion on for first-time customers who sign in online and like her Facebook page. As an incentive you receive $5.00 off your session and taxes are included. This tan was excellent and dried quickly compared to the one at Hollywood Tan – total cost $80.

Another option is signing up with the tanning salon associated with the shows. Absolute Touch is typically the company at the shows. They book you for a tan, are at the show for touch ups right before you go on-stage, and provide the gloss and bikini bite (adhesive to keep your bottoms in place). I did not use this option, but if it is your first show and you've never had a spray tan before, it may be worth it to have some peace of mind knowing if anything happens you can get touched up before you go on stage.

Whatever you do, book your spray tan at least one month in advance to ensure you get the time and day you want. If the show is in a smaller town, the tanning salons may be minimal, so booking early is imperative.

Show gloss – Brand name: Muscle Juice. This is the stuff you pat on right before going out on-stage to give you that shiny look. Although the bottle says spray on, don't! Have your coach spray it on their hands first and then pat it sparingly onto your skin, covering your whole body but highlighting the muscles you want to emphasize ($20 from Hollywood Tan). Caution: You can get docked points for having too much of this on! If you're too shiny, your muscle definition is lost in the bright lights reflecting off of you – I speak from experience.

Hair, makeup and nails – I did my own hair and nails and had my makeup-genius friend, Isabelle, do my makeup for the first show. I only paid for the tools required, which came to $50. To have these things done for you, expect to pay anywhere from $200 or more to get all three done.

Hair removal – For me there was the shave versus wax debate. I conferred with women who had done both and settled on shaving for myself. With the spray tan everything looks uniform, even if you miss a spot! If you have sensitive skin, make sure you wax or shave one or two days before the spray tan – the shaving or waxing bumps can get aggravated by the exfoliation you need to do prior to the spray tan, then as a result are highlighted by the spray when it dries.

Ontario Physique Association (OPA) membership – this membership is valid for one year and allows you to participate in the OPA competitions. It costs $100 and is purchased online, or you can purchase it at some shows at the athletes' registration and pre-show meeting the night before the show. I suggest doing it ahead of time because you have enough to think about the day before.

Show registration fee – this rate varies from $100-125 depending on whether you purchase it early or at the pre-show meeting.

Guests – to attend the show, your supporters will need to pay $25-65 or more depending on whether they are attending the morning show, night show or both. This is the fee for Kitchener and London, but it goes up if your show is in Toronto. The Kitchener show – Oktoberfest – also had VIP seating for $80, which gave guests all day access and reserved seating in the two front rows.

Travel cost – if your show is out of town, account for travel time and expense. You may need a place to stay and transportation, depending on your plans. Often, the show will have an associated hotel with a reduced cost. I had to travel for my second show and decided to stay the night before. The cost of the host hotel was $159 per night. I had friends with me so decided to do an Airbnb. I'm glad I did because, despite the fact that it was a long weekend and the opening for Oktoberfest, I managed to get a townhouse for $100 for the night.

Time off – I worked a half-day the Friday before the competition and took off the Monday after. Other competitors took a week off prior to the competition. It all depends on how fatigued you are and your line of work. For me, being self-employed, there are no sick days and I did better when I focused on patients rather than hunger pangs!

Tallying all of the above, you can get ready for a show in six months to a year, with as little as $2,700 or as much as $8,400. Being fortunate enough to know personal trainers, health care professionals and coaches, really cuts down on costs. Competing in fitness competitions is not only a mental, emotional and physical investment, it is also a major commitment of time and money as well. Make sure you are ready to take the plunge!

Support

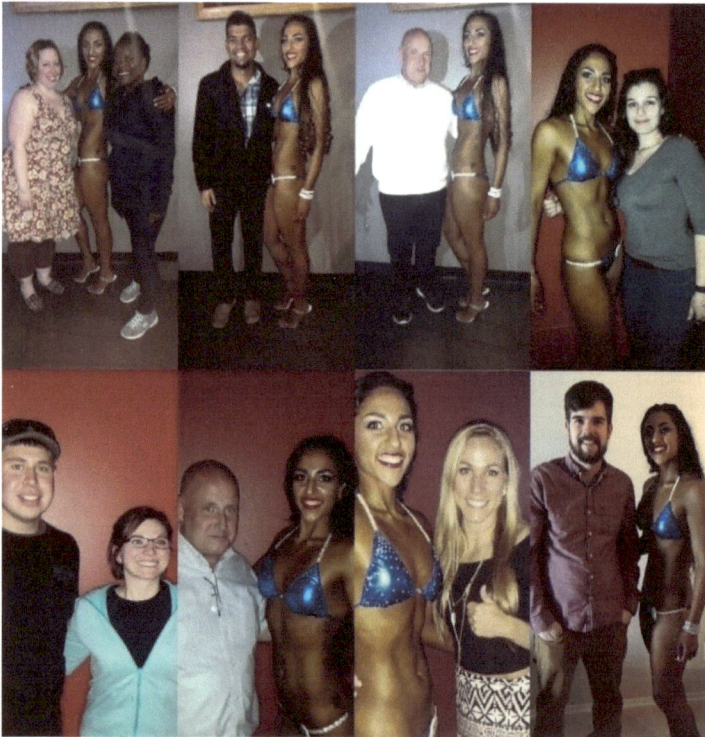

So thankful for family and friends coming to the morning and night shows, May 2017

I was so fortunate to have friends and family excited for me and who supported my new adventure. You need this kind of support because there are times you fall off the wagon, or think you will. There are days when you're tired and grumpy and all you wish for is a burger. You need to vent to sympathetic ears. Past competitors are the best confidants because no matter how long ago their show was, they have vivid memories of their struggle with food.

There may be times when someone says, "Well, all you have to do is eat healthy, what's so hard about that?" Difficult as it may be, try not to bite their head off! Politely explain to them that this is more than the usual healthy eating. This is seeing food as fuel for optimum athletic output. It involves eating only specific foods, in specific amounts and only at specific times. It's like being the only one on food rations, and all that's keeping you there is self-discipline.

Give people a heads-up that you may be tired and irritable at times and have them remind you when this happens. Although you are working hard toward a goal, you don't want to drive your loved ones away in the months preceding the event. Keep in mind you may become a hermit the closer the show gets. It gets harder and harder to resist what is in front of you. So, being two-and-a-half months out from my October 2017 show, I resisted when my dad bought pie, or pizza, or cookies, but in that last month, it was SO hard. You have very few carbs and calories to play with.

Dr. Katelyn Butler-Birmingham

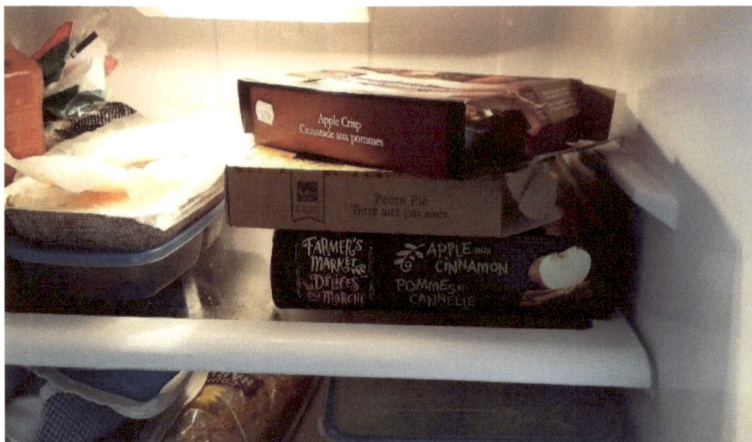

***THREE pies? This is what I'm up against
sometimes...***

I remember the weekend before my show, all I could think about was food – name any kind of sweet thing and I was dreaming about it. My dad keeps these No Name chocolate chip cookies on hand at all times, and I swear I could hear the cookies talking to me. I thought to myself I'll just have one, or two, maybe three. Twenty cookies later I was like OMG how does that happen? But there I was, so happy to be munching away on these cookies that honestly I don't usually even like. In the moment, though, it was the best tasting cookie I'd ever had in my life.

Then came the panic – what have I done, my show is in seven days!! I called my husband in a flurry of guilt, panic and frustration and proceeded to tell him the story of how much I wanted those cookies – no, NEEDED those cookies and that I'd had 20. He's listening intently and then says, "Wait...wait. Roll back a second. Did you just say TWENTY cookies?" "Um, yes," I responded. He burst out laughing, which made me laugh too. Because, who does that? Well, apparently me, while obviously not in my right mind. He assured me it would be okay, that at least I enjoyed it while it lasted, and he still loved me regardless.

Writing this, I realize how crazy it sounds, but while it's happening you see red, so to speak. For me, exactly what I needed then was someone to make light of something I thought was the end of the world. Instead of getting down on me, I just needed to hear someone saying it would be alright and I could start fresh tomorrow.

What Are the Judges Looking For?

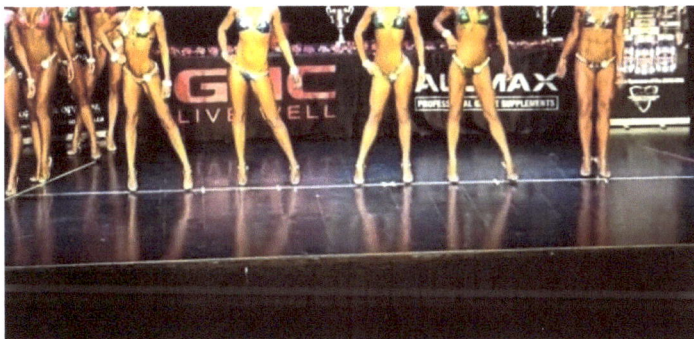

Stephanie Worsfold Show May 2017 – Bikini Medium Lineup – The winner is on the left side of the lineup.

My experience with the judges is mostly in the Bikini category so that will be my main focus. There are other categories for women, such as Figure and Physique. These categories are very different as far as posing and judging criteria. Typically, the women in them are more muscular or have a shorter torso, so not necessarily the hourglass shape. For men, there are Bodybuilding and Physique. Bodybuilding is probably what you are picturing in your head or have seen on TV – it is big muscular men like The Rock or Arnold Schwarzenegger. Physique contestants have less bulk and more tone – the men wear long shorts, look like the typical surfer dude, and their posing is similar to the bikini category.

There are age and height categories to choose from, too. The only category with a weight classification is Bodybuilding. Short is usually 5ft 4in (162.5cm) or less, Medium is over 5ft 4in (162.5cm) to 5ft 6in (167.6cm), Tall is typically over 5ft 6in (167.6cm). If you are registering online and choose the wrong category, don't worry. They do measurements at the competitors' meeting the night before the show so you end up in the right category.

Bikini Specifics

The judges look for the hourglass shape. To emphasize this, they look for well-defined shoulders and glutes – the big round bum. Some judges prefer tight abs, where others prefer a softer look. To impress the judges on the fence, you need to nail your posing.

Although there are two shows, morning and evening, the judges actually decide on the winners during the morning show. They may make some last minute changes at the evening show if, for some reason, the person doesn't show up, but typically they already know who will be in first, second and third places. Having a 'top five' is being phased out, going more toward picking only the top three.

You might be shifted around during the morning show. The judges call your number and have you switch places with another contestant. The order they ask you to stand in has nothing to do with your placing. They move you to compare you more easily to the person beside you. This is where they tease out the finer details of how your physique looks compared to another's.

During a posing class with Melissa Shadd, she relayed a story of a contestant who thought they were in first place because they were first in line and had been called to come out in a line-up twice. The person posted on Instagram that they were winning the show; turns out they didn't. So remember, it is just a comparison. Hold off posting a win until you have the medal!

Each category winner gets a prize, perhaps a gift bag, gym membership, a trip, supplements, etc. Most people want to win a competition so they can go on to the next level to win and get their professional card. This means they have a better chance of a sponsorship and making a career out of competing.

If you don't win a medal, you are still ranked and the scores come out a week after the show. First you are ranked within your height category, then you are given an overall score so you can see how you compared across the entire Bikini category. For my first show, I ranked eighth out of 11 and for the second, I ranked last out of eight competitors in the Bikini Medium Category. It all depends on who shows up that day.

> ...all competitors put in hard work and dedication to their diet and exercise, but also may have used ergogenic aids like caffeine pills, diuretics or even steroids. I'm hoping this information helps natural competitors rise to the top without the negative impact such aids make on the body.

After seeing my photographs, I've been asked a couple of times why I didn't win. Well, it's all about meeting the criteria the judges are looking for with excellent posing. I can point out mistakes I made in both shows, but to the untrained eye it doesn't mean much. I felt so much better about my second show and made some major improvements, which was my goal in entering a second show. As you read this book, factor in that all of the competitors put in hard work and dedication to their diet and exercise, but they may also have used ergogenic aids like caffeine pills, diuretics or even steroids. I'm hoping this information helps natural competitors rise to the top, without the negative impact such aids make on the body. **It is possible to have a completely natural show!**

How Long Does This Take?

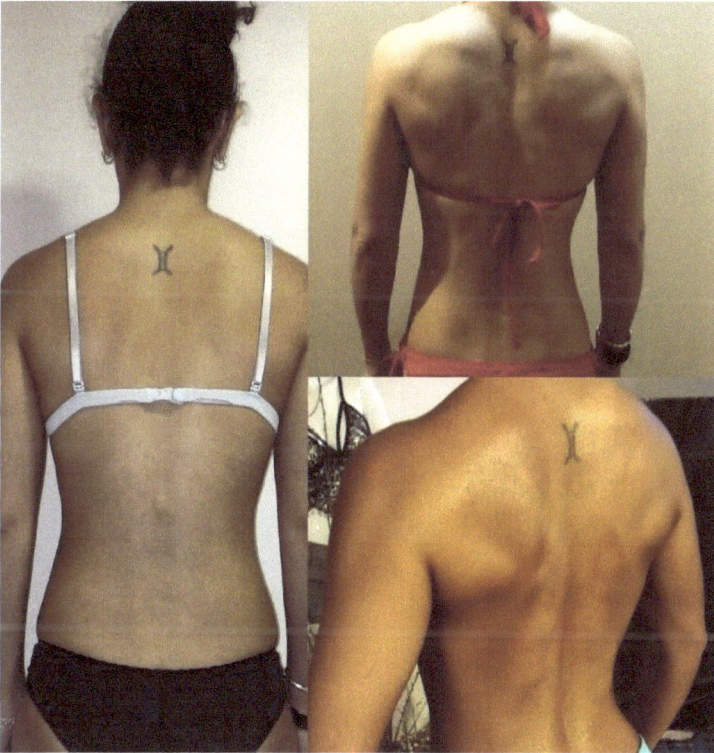

Progress of back – start, middle, end

When preparing for a show, always err on the side of caution and allow more time than you think you need. For my first show, I took five months to prepare. For the second, I took four months. To give you a point of reference, I am in the Bikini Medium category at 5ft 5.5in (166.4 cm). My starting weight was 136 lbs. (61.7 kg) and I ended up at 123 lbs (55.8 kg). If you are measuring body fat percentage along with weight, it is best to be between 10-15% body fat depending on how your body looks and where you tend to carry your weight. For my second show, I started at 146 lbs (66.2 kg) and ended at 129 lbs (58.5 kg). In the Recovery section, see why I jumped from starting at 136 lbs for the first competition to 146 lbs for the next one.

By your second show you know how your body responds and how forgiving it is if you fall off the wagon. Also, at that point, you aren't starting from scratch. You have an excellent muscle base already established and you can tailor your workouts and weight loss accordingly. Healthy weight loss is 1-2 lbs (.450–.900 kg) of body fat loss per week. Keep this in mind and allow for plateaus and unforeseen circumstances. For example, if you have to lose 60 lbs (27.2 kg), allow for at least a year of training and dietary changes. This is a time commitment. I was in the gym for at least two hours six days a week. Sometimes it seems impossible to fit a 30-minute workout in, so take a good hard look at your schedule and see where realistically you can fit in this kind of time commitment.

Pre-Show Meeting

As I mentioned before, there is a mandatory pre-show meeting the night before. This is for any last-minute registration, check-ins, weigh-ins or height measurements depending on your category. The meeting follows. At check-in, you get a pin or button with a number on it. You are called by this number and have to wear it on your suit for the show. It is very important to keep this in a safe spot so you don't lose it. I attached it right away to my suit so I didn't have to think about it the next day.

You need to bring your suit to the meeting because the judges doing the height checks also have a peak at your suit to make sure it is acceptable. There can't be anything hanging off of it, it can't be too small – this is why you need to make sure you get a half-coverage bottom rather than the third-coverage. There are booths offering tanning touchups, pictures and video recordings for the day of the show.

The judges attend and run the meeting. They go over posing, explaining what is expected of you and remind you of arrival times the following day. There are morning and night shows, with a few hours' break in between. The organizers tell you what time to arrive for both. Make sure you also take note of the show's location because it may not be the same as where the meeting is held.

Dr. Katelyn Butler-Birmingham

It is funny to see people at the meeting and then how different they look the next day. Most people show up to the meeting looking very plain – most have just had their tan done and are wearing baggy clothes, no makeup and their hair in a bun. This is in complete contrast to how everyone looks the next day – like total rock stars. The best part about the meeting is the treat bag with samples, shaker bottles and even candy!

Posing

Posing needs special mention here because it is what sets you apart from the other competitors, and places the judges' attention on you. Despite advice to do so, I didn't take posing classes the first time around, so I only found out about the quarter turns the night before the show at the pre-show meeting. They went to the quarter turn because it is more uniform and everyone does the same pose, whereas before you had a handful of poses to choose from and could

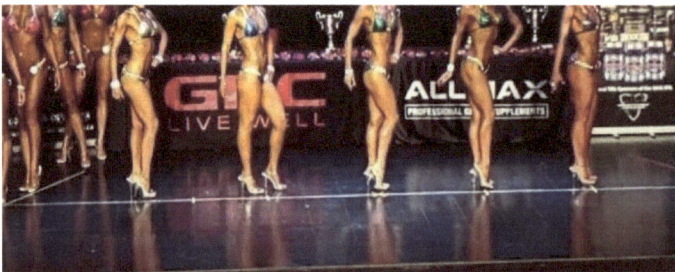

Stephanie Worsfold Show - Bikini Medium lineup – I'm second from left; notice my incorrect straight front leg.

32

choose whichever one made your body type look the best. Needless to say, I was in a panic because all of a sudden, at 9 pm the night before the show, I had to figure out new posing.

June 19, 2017

So the day of the show my coach and I practise ¼-turns the best we can. She went out to watch the girls before my group and came running backstage to tell me that the front leg had to be bent. Well at this point my group is all lined up and I was like, you know what I'm too nervous to change what we practised – I'll just go with this and hope for the best. The knee bent almost had me topple over and I figured I'd rather not fall over on-stage – I don't want to be that memorable! Anyway, I went out and the crowd was going nuts, the music was blaring and they had our group come up. So there I was, focused on footing and smiling – Front pose. Then ¼ turn to the right...the head judge says something...what did he say? Oh well, just keep smiling and posing...and again he repeats. I thought I heard my number but didn't know what the next part was. So I look over at the volunteer who points things out on-stage and guides people where to go. So she puts her hand on her hip and at the same time the judge yells "57, hand on hip!" The crowd gets quiet. Oh shit...that's me for sure – so, flustered, I put my hand on my hip. Then with the back pose same thing – but this time he's talking to 2 of us. Despite being flustered and embarrassed I managed to keep a smile on my face the whole time...my friends and family were there to meet me afterwards and we all had a good laugh about how I got yelled at – definitely something I can only laugh at after the fact.

So, once again – you can win or lose on posing. The competitors' bodies don't look very different, so you need to accentuate your attributes with the posing.

Due to changes within the OPA, they are now moving more toward the International Federation of Body Builders (IFBB) pro league style of posing. This means that, as of January 2018, the quarter turn pose is eliminated from competitions in Ontario. Only front and back poses remain. Count your lucky stars on this because standing in a quarter-turn pose on the sidelines is WAY harder than it looks. I'm guessing this means that comparisons are made easier for the judges and that the Bikini category will need to be a bit more focused on developing abs. You still can rotate your hips in the front pose while keeping your toes pointed forward, but there will be no making up for it with a side pose. Keep up to date with these changes. When you sign up for your OPA card, you will receive e-newsletters. Make sure to read these as they have the most up-to-date information. Also, ensure the posing class you choose is the right one! Stay tuned for more detailed information in the Posing Class section.

What to Bring to the Show

What you bring to the show can really make a difference. A lot of women at the show I went to had full suitcases. I would say a carry-on is too small, but checked luggage is too big. A happy medium is a duffle bag or a medium suitcase with wheels. Beware shoulder bags or backpacks because the straps can make lines in your spray tan! If possible, have your coach or a friend acting as a coach, carry your things.

Here is what you need:
- Makeup for touch ups;
- Eyelash glue;
- 500 ml water;
- Phone;
- Snacks – rice cakes, nut butter, muffin – some had candy, chocolate, potatoes;
- Pocket mirror;
- Gloss spray;
- Flip-flops;
- Exercise band for pre-show pump-up;
- big shirt or robe to put on between shows;
- a change of clothes for afterwards.

Backstage

You soon discover some shows are more organized than others. I did the Stephanie Worsfold Natural Classic in May 2017. The previous venue was always Centennial Hall, but that year it changed to the London Music Hall. Being the first year at the new venue, they were working out some kinks and it will probably be smoother in future years. The volunteers are great for helping you figure out where things are.

Look for postings to tell you what category is first. Most shows have Men's Bodybuilding, then Men's Physique, Women's Physique, Women's Figure and Bikini is last. Determine right away when you're going on, especially if you want to watch part of the show. The Women's Bikini is the big attraction at the end, but Men's Bodybuilding is very entertaining. First they run through their posing routine separately and then they all come out together and do a one-minute *muscle-off*, same idea as a dance-off, but for muscle display. It gets very funny!

Once you know where your name is, look at the two categories before yours so you have plenty of notice to get backstage. Also, take note of the number of people in the preceding categories. The time each category spends on-stage can be fairly short depending on how many people it has. To give you an idea, a category with eight people or less will move very quickly, three to five minutes at most. Some categories only have one person in it, so be mindful that such a category will be over very quickly. A big category has 20 people, which happens in the Bikini category.

Once it gets close to show time, you need time backstage to get ready. Allow at least 20 minutes for your spray shine and then the pre-show pump-up. The pump-up is a series of exercises done to give your muscles a little boost so they look big when you are on-stage. The exercises you choose depend on which muscles you want to emphasize. For example, I did a sequence of push-ups (to perk up my chest and arms), squats, semi-squats and Bulgarian lunges (all for legs and bum), each for 20 reps and three sets. Imagine all of that in five-inch heels! When you do more reps using body weight only, it gets the blood pumping to these muscle groups. The sets allow you to rest that muscle group as you work on another. For example, 20 pushups and then switch to 20 squats. The idea is to get blood flow going without getting sweaty. The exercises you choose to do may be different based on how you look on show day.

Volunteers start calling your category and lining you up by number. The wait in line seemed to take forever. Chatting with the woman in front of me helped pass the time, and knowing everyone was in the same boat, had worked very hard and was ready to step on-stage, eased my nerves.

Show Time!

Take that final deep breath and get that big smile ready! Brace yourself for flashing bright lights, the crowd cheering and music blaring. Remember to breathe and know that this is your moment to show off all your hard work. If you see some people's muscles shaking, that is either from dehydration or nerves. If it is happening to you, just do a slight repositioning.

Although it may seem weird, smile and look directly at the judges. I wanted to look for my friends, but the judges actually want you focused on them. You may have a big group and have to stand on the sidelines while other people are out front doing their posing. Even if this is the case, keep standing in your front pose. You can switch from side to side, but keep smiling and stay in your pose. Although the judges have other people out front, they may still be looking at you.

When it is your row's turn to be in the spotlight, let your posing come naturally. First, the front pose, then quarter-turn to the right (if applicable) so the left side faces the judges, another quarter-turn to the back pose, then quarter-turn so the right side faces the judges, then return to the front pose. Once the initial turns are complete, the judges may have you switch positions with other participants to compare one person to the next, then rank the contestant. They may ask for more turns at this point. Then, before you know it, you're walking off stage and getting ready for the night show!

What Qualifies as Natural Fitness?

Over the years, I've learned that the term *natural* is more of a marketing ploy and catch phrase than anything else. For example, *all natural* soymilk, *all natural* baked cheese crackers, *all natural* fruit smoothie. To me, this use of natural is a joke. I believe completely natural means it comes from the earth and is not altered.

Being a Naturopathic Doctor, I use **natural** healthcare products. The products I recommend come from a plant, but due to their processing they don't fit the above definition of completely natural, unless the

> *To me, natural means it comes from the earth and is not altered.*

whole plant is used – like for a tea. Most of the herbal remedies I use have been distilled to make them more potent – and even that changes how the original plant reacts in the body.

Natural healthcare products can be dangerous, despite them being from plants. Anytime you modify something from its original state, you change how it performs. In later chapters when I discuss caffeine pills and natural fat burners like green tea extract, the importance of this base knowledge becomes clearer. Taking a caffeine pill is very different from chewing a coffee bean, and taking a fat burner is very different from eating green tea leaves. Although they have been made from a plant, their modifications make them completely different from what they were originally. The way we use natural today is like saying that aspirin is natural because it is derived from willow bark – yet it is so far from its original form, with processing and so many additives, that it would be very misleading to call aspirin natural.

Major pressure was put on the over-the-counter-vitamin companies several years ago to clarify what manufacturers were legally allowed to put on their labels. To this day, there is no legislated definition of what natural means for food products other than the fact that companies cannot use the term *natural* if the product contains food colouring, artificial flavours or man-made substances. There is, however, a grey area when it comes to what artificial flavours are. To me, an artificial flavour is one that is fabricated, with some chemicals added to enhance the taste of the product, even if it is isolated from the original item. When the label says natural flavours, it could mean that all or parts of the original product were used.

For example, if you have grapefruit juice that says no artificial flavours have been added, but the label itself says *natural flavouring*, this could be that the grapefruit's essential oil, oleoresin, extract, protein hydrolysate, distillate, or any product of roasting, heating or enzyme fragment, has been used. The interesting thing is, it doesn't even have to come from a grapefruit at all. It could come from any spice, fruit or fruit juice, vegetable or vegetable juice, edible yeast, plant material, meat, seafood, poultry, eggs, dairy products, or fermentation products. This is where food engineering comes in. You could make an *all natural* grapefruit juice with lemon extract, orange distillate and lime resin – all unidentified under the umbrella name *natural flavouring*.

We automatically assume that if something says natural, it is safe or good for us. I, myself, have been guilty of picking up the light blue or green packaged container of some product and not reading the label to see what changes were made to the original product supposedly to make it healthier. Was artificial no-calorie sweetener added, or was it made with natural versus artificial flavours? My advice to you is, if you want to do this show naturally, define what that means to you. Will you do everything with food and water alone? Will you use ergogenic aids? Whatever you decide, make sure to weigh the risk to benefit ratio and know the short- and long-term consequences of choosing certain products.

For me, doing a natural show means using food, water and protein powder. The protein powder filled in any gaps and ensured I was getting enough protein without exceeding my calorie allowance for the day. I trust the brand I use because it was third-party tested, but if natural to you means only food and water, find a coach who will tailor a plan like that just for you. There is no reason a show can't or shouldn't be done with food and water alone.

Dr. Katelyn Butler-Birmingham

PART II: The Practical

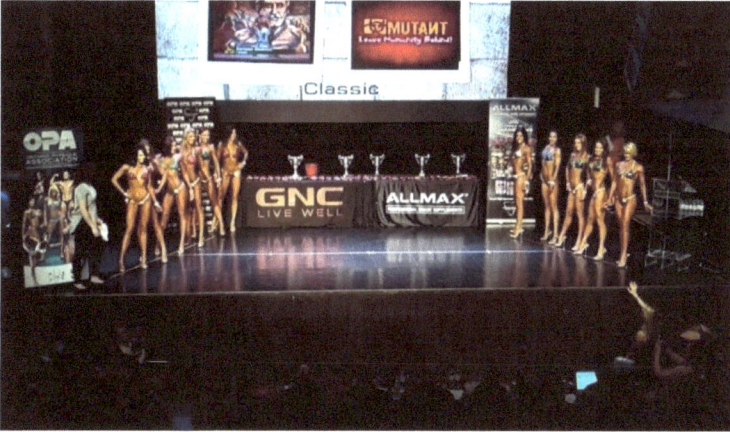

Stephanie Worsfold Natural Classic – May 2017

"You need to love yourself; you are number one. If you don't love yourself, you can't truly love anyone else."

– Peter Birmingham,
my Dad and the fittest man I know

Body Image

Now that you've gone over everything you need to know to get organized for your first show, and it seems doable, we need to stop and talk about the uncomfortable for a moment.

One of my aunts is a therapist so I already know what she would say on the topic. If you have any body image issues or have struggled with an eating disorder, DO NOT do a competition until you have addressed these things. I must say, I agree. If you know of something pre-existing, it is best to address it before proceeding. Unfortunately, there are many competitors who feel they have a healthy relationship with food – myself included – only to discover, after the fact, that the rebound weight gain brings on some surprising emotions.

> *If you have any body image issues or have struggled with an eating disorder, DO NOT do a competition until you have addressed these issues.*

I've heard several competitors talk about the rebound weight gain and how it made them feel. The most common stories are of periods of depression that followed and lasted anywhere from three weeks to a year. Most women weren't fully prepared for the rebound weight gain. For some others, it was part of the post-competition let-down.

Let's first take a look at the post-competition let-down. Competition day is like a wedding day. You want everything to be perfect – perfect tan, perfect hair, perfect nails and makeup. All your family and friends have been cheering you on along the way and they are there, part of this big event. Only winners go on to the next level; for everyone else, there's all this excitement and then suddenly, it's over. Some people get very discouraged if they don't do well. They've worked so hard for a long time to get on that stage.

I can tell you, my first show was not great. Initially, I was flustered about how it went, but then it drove me to search for another show so I could do better. If looking forward to something great coming up helps, or you want the challenge of improving, pick yourself up as best you can and go on to the next!

Every show is totally different. The competitors change and you have a chance to get better in areas that held you back. Maybe your posing needs some work. If you want to know exactly what you need to work on, you can purchase a voice recording of the head judge critiquing your performance. This service is sold at the athletes' meeting, so there's nothing to worry about ahead of time and it makes it possible to learn exactly what the judges thought. Once you know what held you back, focus on perfecting that factor.

The biggest thing to keep in mind is that how you do in your first show doesn't impact how you do in the second, or any other. The winner of each category is chosen by comparing you with other competitors right in that moment. Don't be discouraged. If you enjoy the show, challenge yourself to another.

As mentioned, the second biggest concern impacting competitors is the rebound weight gain. Your coach is very knowledgeable about this, so listen to what they say. Mine told me that people typically gain all their weight back within two weeks. I heard the words, but it didn't compute; not until I experienced it myself.

The first time around, I gained back all my weight and then some. When prepping for the show I was hyper-aware of my body and how it looked, constantly checking measurements or posing to see what work still needed to be done. After my first show, I threw caution to the wind eating whatever I wanted for a month, not paying attention at all to how I looked. Three weeks after the show I remember carrying my treatment table – something I do all the time – up the stairs at the office and being out of breath. I got to the top of the stairs, put the table down and was thinking, "What is happening?" That's when it really hit me. The free-for-all eating had to stop.

I looked my best on competition day, but you only look that small for one or two days.

That night I looked at myself and didn't like what I saw. I wondered if people at the clinic or at the gym noticed how big I'd gotten. And when I say big, I mean ten pounds over my starting weight. Objectively that isn't much, but subjectively it seemed huge. After talking about this with colleagues and close friends, I realized no one had noticed. They thought I had gained five pounds maybe, but not twenty. I was incredibly relieved at how little they focused on my weight.

At the same time, it was scary and gave me a real personal view of what people who suffer with eating disorders go through every day. It rendered me speechless because I never would have expected that from myself. I had compassion for those diseases before; now I have empathy. It is such a lonely place to be when you are the only one who sees something and, no matter what others say, you see what you see.

For my second show I was much more aware and prepared for the post-competition weight gain. So, although when I look at pictures I can hardly believe I was really that small, I remind myself that I looked my best on competition day, but you only look that small for one or two days. Once you start rehydrating, it doesn't even have to be eating, you

Preparing for a show naturally is important if you want to mitigate rebound weight gain. Taking months instead of weeks to prepare means fewer food restrictions and a healthier weight-loss rate that's more sustainable in the long term.

notice your body holds on to everything. I will explain why later.

Another key thing to remember is that to compete you conform to a specific definition of beauty and fitness. The criteria judges look for are very specific and attainable for only short periods of time. Once the show is over, you have to come back to reality – the reality where you eat out occasionally, use sauces and drink lots of water!

Taking your time to prepare for a show and doing it naturally is so important if you want to mitigate the rebound weight gain. Taking months to prepare versus weeks means you don't undergo so many food restrictions, you lose weight at a healthy and safe pace, and your weight loss is more sustainable.

If you continuously cycle through weight loss and weight gain, as yo-yo dieters do, it becomes harder and harder to lose weight. Our bodies have evolved to store energy sources, primarily as fat. Due to many famines across generations, our bodies have become very good at holding on, especially when they are pushed as they are with physical training or periods when nutrients are limited.

Going from starvation to having plenty on numerous occasions, makes your body decide, "Hey, I need to stock up because I don't know when the next famine, AKA diet, is going to happen." So instead of shedding weight, the body holds on to everything you put into it for later use.

Taking your time and using whole foods and water to get ready for a show, decreases your restrictions during the cutting phase and you won't make your body artificially smaller than it can naturally achieve. This minimizes more extreme rebound weight gain, and gives you the confidence to know your body's true capabilities, and its limits.

Competitions Naturally

"Today I will do what others won't, so tomorrow I can accomplish what others can't."

- Jerry Rice

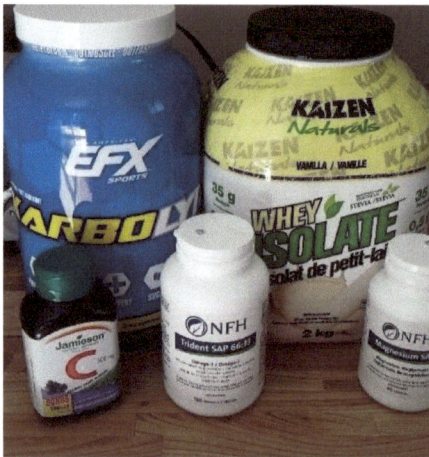

Supplements I used for the first show

In the photo above, you see the supplements I used along my journey. I dropped the Karbolyn altogether for my second show and was down to the bare minimum of fish oil, magnesium, vitamin C and protein powder. Although I'm not a fan of Karbolyn, its benefit is that you get pure carbs without the added calories of having a piece of fruit. Whatever you do, DO NOT use a full scoop of Karbolyn. It gives a major sugar rush and likely too many calories from carbohydrates. Ensure you use the right amount for you. If, instead, you truly want to use food only as fuel, drop the use of Karbolyn. Kaizen is third-party tested and has few ingredients, which is great. All in all, you have to pick what is right for you. You don't have to use any adjuncts if you don't want to. Tell your coach; they will figure out a way to deliver a plan that fits with what you want.

I was naïve getting into the fitness competition world, thinking competitors looked like that just from diet and exercise. Looking back, I don't know why I thought that. Now that I know what supplements are allowed in a *Natural* show, the notion of everyone at the shows using only diet and exercise to meet their goals seems foolish. Green tea extract, conjugated linoleic acid (CLA), and garcinia cambogia are the most popular fat burners. People think they are harmless

> *Putting yourself through something rigorous shouldn't compromise your health or safety.*

because they are made from natural sources like plants and, in CLA's case, the fat found in grass fed beef and butter. **Natural does not mean safe.** Many herbs interact with medications, are easily overdosed, or cause allergic reactions.

In recent years, natural healthcare products have undergone scrutiny, especially vitamins and protein powders. There were concerns that the ingredients in the product did not match the label and that fillers were the main ingredients. Fillers are the binding agent of the pill – what keeps it together – and generally are chemically engineered to take up space in the pill, to change its colour, shape or texture. Since then, tightened labelling and testing regulations have things on track. However, unless a company has a natural health product number, meaning their supplements or herbs have undergone rigorous clinical trials to ensure safety, effectiveness and third-party testing, you can't be sure what you are buying. Products sold at health food and body-building supply stores don't guarantee this kind of testing.

When you use a **fat burner**, whether from a plant or not, you are altering the body's normal function. That's why rebound weight gain occurs when you stop taking the supplement. Also it is artificially making your body smaller than it would normally be with just food, water and exercise. I had one woman tell me that her body type is naturally more muscular and after getting so thin with diuretics and fat burners, she has never felt the same since. Her strength isn't what it was and even her body shape has changed. Putting yourself through something rigorous shouldn't compromise your health and safety. You still need to feel comfortable in your skin once the competition is over.

So, remember these three things: "natural" doesn't necessarily mean safe; expect additional rebound weight gain when discontinuing use of fat burners; and, only use tested products. To be sure what you are taking is safe, consult with a Naturopath. They know about interactions between drugs and herbs.

> **The take-home message here is threefold:**
> 1. **just because it says natural doesn't mean it is safe;**
> 2. **when you use fat burners, expect some rebound weight gain when you discontinue them; and,**
> 3. **only use tested products if using any at all.**

I thought **steroid** use had gone out the window, especially with the widely available information on the consequences users suffer. And then there's the seemingly obvious – why take steroids if you are in a Natural competition? However, I know of someone who did, so using steroids is still in practice. Probably because there are ways now to filter it out of your system in a week, so it doesn't show up on the urine test when you are at the show.

I am committed to all-natural training, so although I am told rapid filtering works, I was not interested in learning how. Random tests are done at the shows and looking at some of the athletes you can tell they have taken steroids, but nothing can be proven.

Using steroids is more popular than you may think, even for people not training for fitness competitions. I have a colleague who is a chiropractor and has had several patients ask not to be touched in a certain area because it is their steroid injection site. The most popular steroids are injectables that contain growth hormone. Growth hormone is naturally produced in the body, and in a healthy person is at the level they need. The injected synthetic version is over and above what is needed and is part of the component that makes muscle tissue grow artificially. After only one use of steroids, muscle tissue is forever changed.

One use of steroids changes how muscles respond and how they grow (hypertrophy). Due to the nature of the injectable synthetic steroid, you run into the same cautions and dangers posed by other drugs. For example, you must ensure the steroid is not mixed with anything, the injection technique is safe, and you are using the proper dose. In addition, be aware of the associated side effects of taking steroids, such as extreme anger, mood swings, heart attack, and impotence, to name a few.

> *After one use of steroids, your muscle response is forever changed.*

Diuretics, like steroids, are fairly commonplace in Natural shows. Diuretics are not a benign drug. They are used to treat high blood pressure and are also known as 'water pills'. They work by getting salt to come out in the urine. The salt automatically pulls water with it thus taking water out of your system. Lowering the system's amount of fluid helps to lower blood volume, which in turn lowers blood pressure.

Why, you ask, would an athlete who presumably has a healthy blood pressure want to take these? Because of the pill's mechanism of action – by pulling water out of your system, you are shedding water weight, especially if you're limiting your water intake. This gives athletes an edge because they look even more toned and tight.

However, like any other medication, diuretics have side effects. Taking too much, could take excessive salt out of the system, causing dizziness, headaches, dehydration, nausea and muscle cramps. You are already in a dehydrated state for the show because of the *drying out phase* that we will talk about later. Adding a diuretic to the mix can have serious consequences. If you worry about passing out on stage from the pre-show jitters, now you have an added worry; passing out from a bottoming out blood pressure, or worse, a cardiac event.

Some contestants use **caffeine pills** for a boost of energy. When eating a very clean diet – meaning a diet without dairy, grains, simple sugar, alcohol or caffeine – even the slightest amount of caffeine, whether it be from chocolate, green tea, black tea, coffee, Coke, etc., can give you a caffeine buzz. Most caffeine pills contain 200-300 mg of caffeine. A cup of coffee (250 ml) has around 100-150 mg of caffeine, depending on how it is prepared. Looking at the numbers you're probably thinking, okay, so if I drink two coffees before work I'm probably getting the equivalent of a caffeine pill every day. BUT, it takes time for you to drink the coffee. It's not just an immediate shot of 250 mg of caffeine at once. A caffeine pill can really amp you up within about 15 minutes.

Think back to a time you overdosed on coffee, if you ever have done so. What followed? The jitters, anxiety, heart pounding, sweating, restlessness, racing thoughts – one caffeine pill can do that to your system. I don't recommend these for anyone, but especially for anyone with anxiety, high blood pressure, caffeine sensitivity, a heart condition, panic attacks or those who have never had coffee before.

Don't get me wrong, there will be days when you are dragging yourself to the gym, or are so carb depleted that your energy is basically non-existent, but if you are feeling really low, use a small black coffee or tea. This helps you avoid any pill side effects and avoids the chemically engineered fillers used to make the pills.

Self-Care

When you get into the full swing of training and your meal plan, it's very easy to ignore small hurts here and there. Training should be a fun experience and you should not have to be in pain. This plays into taking the time you need to safely and effectively meet your goals. If you are prone to injury, or are starting from a place with

Taking care of yourself, and taking rest days when you need them, keeps you from falling apart, literally.

muscle imbalances, or significant weight loss is needed, self-care is extremely important. I have a history of not being the most compliant patient, but I quickly realized that had to stop. If you want to keep training at a high level, eat well, work, go to school etc., you need to address things as they come up, whether they be mental or physical.

For me that meant from the outset of training being cautious of some old injuries: a second degree tear of my right hamstring in 2013; whiplash, concussion and elbow injuries from a car accident in 2014; and, a first degree tear of my left hamstring in 2014. Although these are a few years old, I still feel them every so often. When I first started training I couldn't run for more than a couple of minutes before my neck was completely out of whack. Also, I need to warm up for 10-15 minutes before doing leg exercises or sprints, and I have to stretch my legs after any kind of workout. My workouts had to be tailored with this in mind.

June 19, 2017
A week and a half before the competition – literally Wednesday, May 3rd, 2017, I woke up and bounced out of bed ready to start my day and something happened. I could feel a nagging in my lower back on the left side. I went to the gym as usual and carried on with my day. After seeing a few patients, my back stiffened up to the point where I couldn't even move my neck without feeling a sharp pain down the left side of my back. I told myself to keep calm – maybe this would all be better in the morning. NOPE. I woke up Thursday morning and it was even worse. I could barely get out of bed. The competition was May 13th, 2017. I had 10 days to get better. I went to work early that day to see if I could get in for a massage and chiropractic. As I got out of my car I got a sharp pain, which gave me a hint that the back pain was actually stemming from my glutes. Sure enough, I found a bunch of trigger points in my left glute and pressing on them gave me a bit of relief... 3 chiropractic and 4 massage visits later, and a lot of stretching and Epsom salt baths... I was feeling about 95% by Friday, May 12th, 2017. Now keep in mind my workouts have been down the drain because of the pain. So, all I was really doing was walking. When the day finally came, I think I was running on adrenaline, nerves and excitement because my back felt normal and I was good to walk in my five-inch heels.

I'm lucky that I have the knowledge that I do about my past injuries, my muscle imbalances and anatomy, because before even going to the chiropractor I had a good idea of what was going on. Generally, I would suggest you avoid self-diagnosing; Google can be a scary place. Despite working on my muscle imbalances and stretching it just wasn't enough for my training level. It is hard to see yourself, so to prevent injury, have a full assessment done before you go hard at the gym. Have someone who focuses in Sports Medicine assess your posture, gait, arches, muscle imbalances, and treat current or previous injuries. Addressing where you are starting from helps you maximize your workouts and prevent injury along the way.

My Healthcare Team

Karen Alexander, Personal Trainer/Coach
Dr. Elisha Cook, Doctor of Naturopathy
Michaela Elliot, Registered Massage Therapist
Saadiya Ghanem, Personal Trainer
Dr. Zenin Haji, Doctor of Chiropractic
Dr. Shawn Martin, Doctor of Chiropractic
Monica Seabra, Registered Massage Therapist
Chris Smith, Registered Massage Therapist
Myself, Doctor of Naturopathy, Training Athlete

It is best to have more than one practitioner in each area for a couple of reasons. If your schedule is all over the place, or your regular practitioner is booked at the time you want, you have a backup and less of an excuse to ignore whatever is bothering you.

Hard workouts and cleaning up your diet at the same time have a combined saving grace. More than just muscle wasting is at stake when you eat poorly and try to workout at a high intensity. The immune system takes a beating when you amp up your workouts to one- to two-hour sessions, six days a week.

There are two extremes of the exercise continuum: not doing any physical activity at all, which increases your risk of chronic disease; and, working out a lot, and having your risk of acute illness or injury go up significantly. The best example is the marathon runner who gets a terrible cold that turns into bronchitis the day after their race. Working out is a stress on the body. That is why the recovery days and sleep are so important.

Looking at it physiologically, in stressful situations your body releases a hormone called cortisol. The stressful situation could be that you slept through your alarm and are stuck in traffic on the way to an exam, or it could be that you are pushing yourself to the max during a workout. In both of these situations, cortisol is being released. An excess of cortisol has many negative side effects, but the one most easily noticed is its suppressive effect on the immune system. Chronically elevated cortisol can impair immune function, meaning you are more susceptible to disease, including colds and flus.

For Blood Donors

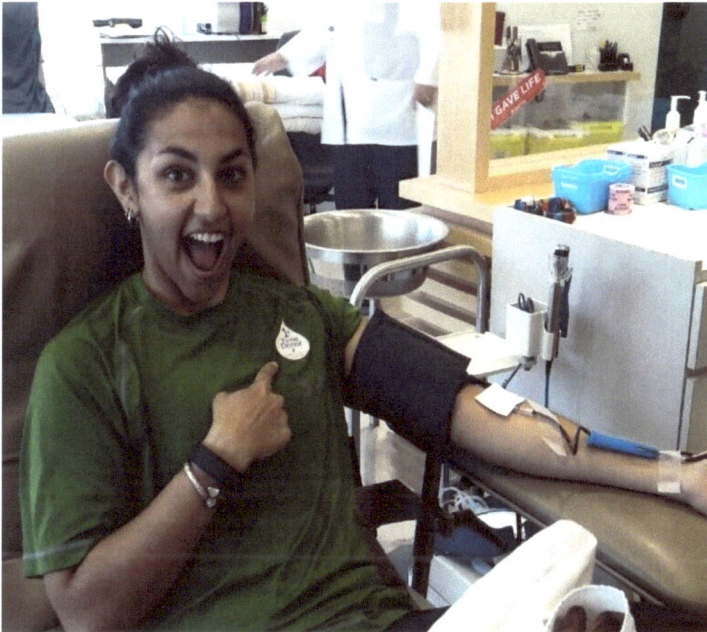

***My first time donating blood – very excited about
getting my sticker that said so***

I've wanted to donate blood for a very long time, but
tattoos along the years have kept me from doing so. I
would have been able to do it earlier this year, but
decided to wait to see how my first competition went,
especially because I was told I would be tired from
the lack of calories and carbs. As I headed into my
second competition I was aware of what made me
tired and recognized the signs in my body. My good
friend, Yasmine, donates on a regular basis, so we

61

Dr. Katelyn Butler-Birmingham

decided to go together the next time she was due. We recruited two other friends to join us as well.

If you're wondering about donating blood, I found it a very pleasant experience and highly recommend it. From walking in the door to when we left it took about an hour. It was neat to find out that just that one donation can save three people's lives. All you need is to show some ID, fill out a questionnaire and they check your haemoglobin, temperature and blood pressure. Then you're all set. It seemed odd having so many people concerned about whether I felt faint. I've never fainted in my life, so wasn't worried that would happen.

There was a small poke when the needle went in, but then I didn't feel it at all. I was a little concerned when my first three fingers went numb about halfway through, but apparently that is a normal occurrence. I didn't like looking at the tube and watching blood coming out of my arm, but looking at others' was okay. I also learned that people get competitive with how fast they can fill the bag and that the Emergency Medical Services (EMS), Ontario Provincial Police (OPP), Royal Canadian Mounted Police (RCMP), London Police and Firefighters all have a competition going to see which group donates the most. The RCMP was winning at the time I was donating. After the donation was complete I was invited to sit in the reception area and got free juice and snacks.

I donated July 29th, 10 weeks from the Oktoberfest competition. You are advised to avoid heavy lifting for a couple of days after donating, so I made sure to do an arm day the day before the donation. I went on a short hike the day of the donation and did a leg day the day after. After the donation I felt great, had lunch with the donation crew then went home and took an hour nap – I was pretty tired. I didn't have any bruising or soreness in my arm the day of the donation. That night my arm felt a bit tight, like I wanted to keep it bent, but that was all.

Sunday, the day after the donation, I felt great – my usual self, ready to hit the gym hard. Monday I was tired and didn't want to get out of bed. I still did a chest and calf workout, but by the end of it I was toast. I did half the intensity for my cardio, and that trend continued for the week. I took Friday off to see if that would help. All in all, it took about five days to fully recover from the donation. The odd feeling in my donation arm also resolved within those five days.

> *If you are a blood donor, or considering becoming one while training, I suggest donating 2½ months before or shortly after the show.*
>
> *It took me about 5 days to recover.*

If you are a blood donor, or are considering becoming one while training, my best suggestion is to do the last donation two and a half months before the show or shortly thereafter – before you start eating all the junk food you ever wanted.

The Spray Tan

I believe the spray tan needs its own section because if you've never had one before, there are so many small details to know! Make sure you follow the directions provided by the tanning salon very closely because even a wrong choice in clothing colour can ruin your tan.

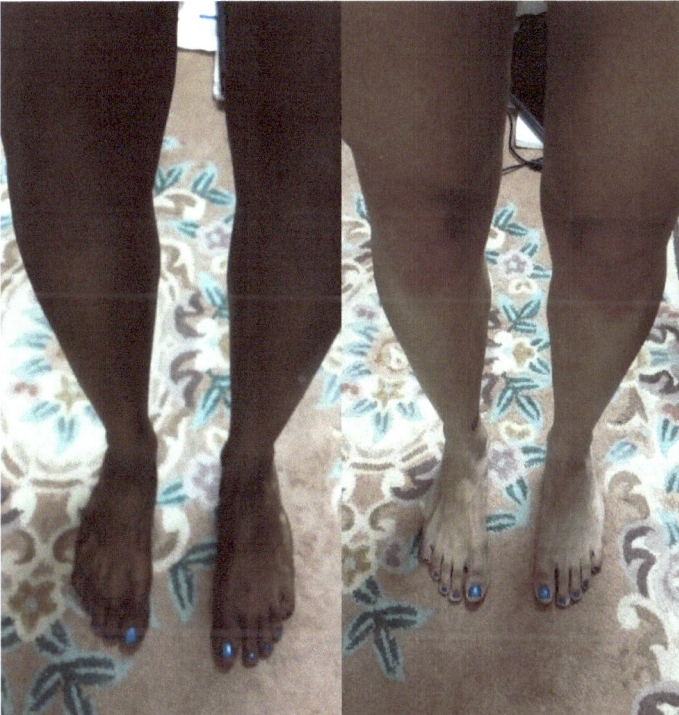

First spray tan at Hollywood Tan in London, ON –
After (left) and Before (right)

Dr. Katelyn Butler-Birmingham

DO:	DO NOT:
Ask specifically for a Fitness Competition Spray Tan.	Shower after the tan – water/sweat will make your tan run.
Book well in advance – at least one month.	Wear deodorant – your armpits will turn yellow/green.
Have the tan done the night before the show.	Wear red clothing – the dye mixes with the tanning solution and you turn green.
Shower before the tan using a loofah or scrub to exfoliate the skin.	Have tight clothing, zippers or buttons.
Shave prior to the tan, but if waxing, have it done 1-2 days before the tan.	Put anything on your skin after the pre-tan shower. Avoid lotions, creams, salves etc.
Dry completely before putting on any clothing.	While you are drying, wear or touch anything that you are afraid to stain.
Wear flip-flops and a big T-shirt or silky robe post tan.	Be shy. You're wearing nothing but a shower cap at the tan.
If you can, have someone drive you to and from the tanning parlour so you can focus on not touching anything.	Sleep naked after the tan.
Use a Dixie® cup to pee – cut a hole in the bottom of the cup and use it as a funnel to prevent streaking your tan with any potential backsplash.	Forget to throw your Dixie® cup in the garbage after use.

I wanted my room to be cool at night because it was necessary to wear a loose fitting long-sleeved shirt and loose pants as well as socks on my hands. Ensure the clothing is not red because the red dye can mix with the spray-tan solution and turn your tan green. Cotton is the best material. It is breathable and won't stick to your tanned skin. Do not wear Under Armor®. Although this brand of clothing is known for its ability to wick sweat, it is not good for post-tan use because it creates a damp environment making the tan dry more slowly, which means it has more potential to streak. The socks on your hands keep you from touching your face and leaving hand prints on it. I didn't want to stain my sheets either, so I put an old sheet down and slept on top of that. This sounds uncomfortable and it is, but you probably won't sleep that well anyway, since it is the night before the show!

What I didn't expect was for the spray tan to stain my nails. To prevent this, you can either have your nails painted when you leave the tanning place, or repaint them after the spray to cover any staining. For time's sake, you may need to do your nails before the tan; just know the spray tan will be on them too.

It took about two hours for my tan to dry. My skin is like a sponge, so it really took in the spray tan. You may not take as long to dry. If you're like me and you've written a note on your hand that takes three days to come off, no matter how many times you wash your hands, then you are likely a little sponge too. There are a few suggested ways to take the tan off when the show is over. Lemon juice and baking soda seem to be the most popular. I didn't use either, just soap and water and it took about two weeks to come off completely but, again, my skin is a sponge. For most people it comes off in about a week. Another suggestion from Shoreline Glow tanning was to soak in baby oil for as long as possible, take a hot bath and use a loofah to scrub it off your skin.

Most people are afraid to touch anything after their

After-Spray-Tan Etiquette
- *Always wipe down the toilet seat after use.*
- *Always discard any paper cups used to prevent pee splash.*

spray tan, but once you're dry, you may forget about it momentarily. However, here is some spray tan etiquette to remember: always wipe down the toilet seat (The person who comes in after you will wonder why the seat is brown. Don't make them wonder, just wipe it down!); and, if you use a Dixie® cup to prevent pee splash, make sure to throw it in the garbage. You don't want to be the person who clogs the toilet!

If, for peace of mind, you book with Absolute Touch, be prepared for them to book your tan at their convenience. You are not notified of what time your tan will be until the Wednesday before the show, provided your show is that Saturday. They also book touch-ups, which can be any time before you go on stage. That means it may be booked at some point between the morning and evening show. This is important because if you had plans to leave the venue right after the morning show, you may have to change those plans. If you miss your scheduled touch-up, there may not be another time to fit you in, especially because they have everyone booked back-to-back. I much prefer to book my own tans because I know exactly when they are and I can leave right after my category is done on stage. You may ask why this would be important. For me, it was because I opted to take naps between both shows, something I highly recommend. It keeps you from thinking about food or dry mouth and you feel refreshed for Round 2!

May 26, 2017
So the spray tan...having a permanent tan myself, I was skeptical about needing one, but one of my colleagues at the gym who has competed and has a similar skin tone had it done, so I just went with it. Ultimately, I'm glad I did. Karen told me I'd be naked for this thing, but jeez you are seriously fricking NAKED! All you have on is this shower cap. So, I get there early and they take me back to this room – well more like a closet. The walls are copper except for one wall that's covered by a huge mirror. The woman tells me to take everything off and put the shower cap on. Okay good... that's done. They put a housecoat over my bag and clothes. Am I supposed to put this thing on? Hmm. She didn't say I should. Alright, well here I am, completely naked.

When is she coming back? Am I just supposed to stand here. What should I do with my hands. Hands on hips. No. Hands behind back. No. Umm. Arms crossed. No. I eventually settle on hands clasped in front of me. I'm not sure how long that went on for, but eventually she came back and then the first thing she asks me is if this is my first tan. Jeez – is it that obvious? Yes. Probably is.

She turns on the machine, which seems very loud, and asks me to stand with my feet hip-width apart and my hands up. The spray feels cool. It's a good thing I worked out my shoulders, because you have your arms up all the time – you can't have them touch your body at all. Everything is going fine on the front. Then she tells me to move my feet further apart and turn my foot out. Everything is out there now. It's almost worse to have the mirror across from you because you can't even kid yourself about how exposed you may or may not be. Then comes the ultimate 'out there' part...She tells me to turn around...and then to bend over. OMG. What? You have to bend at the waist and her face is literally at butt height. This is where you have to hope you don't let one go. Anyway after a few more bends and turns it was finally over, then comes the drying.

She had to go to another client, so she asked if I would mind if her boss came to check on me. Why not? This person has seen every possible angle of my body, what's one more person seeing me just standing here? The appointment was for 4 pm, and I was there until 6:10 pm and I still wasn't dry. They had three fans around me – still with my arms up. But I had to get to registration, so that was that!

Posing Class

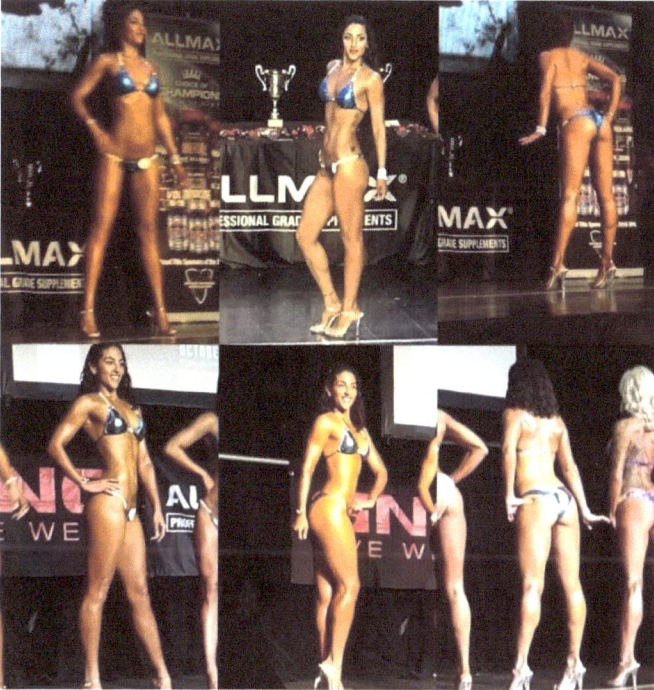

***Comparison of posing from Show 1 to Show 2 – the
mistakes I made in the first show are glaringly
obvious now, but only after taking a posing class!***

As mentioned previously, I did not take posing
classes for my first show, but after the fact, sincerely
wished I had. I wasn't about to make that mistake
again, so decided to take posing classes for the
second show. The Kitchener show is organized by
one of the OPA judges and she also runs a posing

class. If you can find a judge who teaches a class, choose this! They have the most up-to-date information, as well as being able to provide you with tips on what they look for and common mistakes. Needless to say, I learned a lot taking a class with judge Melissa Shadd in Kitchener, Ontario!

Some posing tips and mistakes are included below.

Tips

Think of being on stage as your job, a very short-lived job after all your preparation, but make sure you are focused.

1) Practise posing daily the whole month before the show, at least 10-15 minutes, twice a day.
2) Practise holding each pose to help with endurance so you don't fidget on stage. I used a timer and started at 30 seconds, working my way up to three minutes.

> *I did not take posing classes for my first show, but sincerely wished I had.*
>
> *If you can find a judge who teaches a posing class, choose this!*

3) Practise smiling the ENTIRE time you're practising posing. It's not often that you smile for 10 minutes straight, so you need endurance there too.
4) When you're on the sidelines on stage, keep posing and smiling like you're at centre stage. The judges are still looking at you!

Being told to practise smiling sounds strange, but I want to stress it's important to smile all the time you are on stage. Even if you feel silly doing it, it looks great to the judges and the audience. If you don't practise, your face can start twitching and your smile looks like it has an electric current flowing through it – not particularly attractive and even slightly off-putting.

Always look at the judges. This was strange to me, so I didn't for much of the first show. It seemed more natural to look at the crowd and smile at them, but it isn't the crowd who picks the winner, so smile your heart out at the judges because they are the ones to please.

Common Mistakes

Melissa Shadd tells you that every show has someone who does one of the following. Although the judges see it all the time, don't let it be you!

1) Someone crashes into the person in front of them, generally due to distraction, such as being excited to hear your family and friends' cheering and looking for them in the crowd rather than paying attention. Watch what you are doing.
2) Bending too far forward while in your back pose points the wrong things at the judges. Instead, stick out your bum while keeping your torso upright.
3) Bending your legs in the front and back pose, when the only time one knee is supposed to be

73

bent is for the side pose. Keep them straight otherwise.

4) Arms in the wrong position while in your back pose. Remember, one hand is on the hip, the other arm is straight with the wrist up like on a "Barbie" doll.

5) Torso facing the wrong way. Always turn your torso so that your shoulders face the judges.

6) Toes pointing out or in, or one foot in front of the other. In all poses, your feet need to be parallel, toes pointing forward.

The hardest things for me to remember were to stand up tall in my back pose and not squeeze my shoulder blades together. Squeezing them squishes the back up, and takes away from your hard work. In the relaxed position, the overall muscle definition is seen much better. The other concern was sufficient flexibility in my torso to have my shoulders rotated enough for them to be facing the judges in front and side poses. I practised a lot in the mirror. I suggest from two weeks out you practise without one so you can feel the pose; try to feel when you're coming out of it. Even better is to record yourself or practise with your coach until you can self-correct.

Short Term Vacation Prep

If you decide to do a show several months down the road, and are taking your time to lose weight, you may want to look at all the events you have planned between then and now. I started training for my first show on December 19th, 2016. I didn't exactly plan that out well because Christmas was literally around the corner. But it really focused me on what I was putting into my body and how much. Don't get me wrong, I still had Christmas and New Year's dinners, but just one plate

I recommend announcing to your friends that you have limited cheat meals, and if they want to share those with you, they need to book them in advance.

and no dessert. Getting closer to March, people start coming out of hiding from winter and want to go out. So there are always those impromptu things that come up, as well. For such occasions I recommend announcing to your friends that you have limited cheat meals, and if they want to share those with you, they need to book them in advance. I remember one month I was booking six weeks in advance.

My second show had a double whammy. First, I had a short stay in Toronto at the World Fitness Expo, heading back home for a day to play in a soccer tournament. Then, I was off to Hawaii.

Here is what you need to do for a short term stay:

1) Prepare all of your meals ahead of time;
2) Pack extra snacks in case you are delayed at any time;
3) Have a cooler or lunch box;
4) Have multiple freezer packs;
5) Ensure all of your food is cooked right through in case you are at a place that has no microwave or fridge.

It is a lot of work at first, but you get used to prepping two or three days' worth of food for your regular routine. I spent about two hours on Sundays getting meals ready for the week. What I prepared lasted three to four days. That was the bulk of my food, then there were just last minute veggies or nut butters to add. When you start running low on lean proteins, marinate your meat or fish and then cook it the following day. Overall, you really save time and well might use this method of getting things done all in one shot even after the show is done.

August 21, 2017
So let me start with TO. That was a one-day trip. I followed my own advice and packed food, did great all day, except for the last meal. I was stuck in a meeting and ravenous. They gave us 'healthy' snacks – protein bars and organic coconut clusters. Lucky for me two of the three protein bars had almonds, but I devoured the one protein bar I could eat and the coconut clusters – definitely 300 calories

over budget. On the bright side, despite having an entire day of lectures I still walked between classes and managed to log 12,088 steps on my Fitbit.

Just to give you a little context, I'm allergic to almonds – hence my gratefulness that two of the three bars contained them so I couldn't eat them. All in all, the unexpected can throw the best plans awry. I wasn't planning on being in that last meeting so long and with no microwave in sight. SO, the lesson here is, always have a contingency plan. In hindsight, I should have packed a handful of cashews to tide me over. But this is what it's all about – seeing where the weak spots are in your meal plan and correcting them for the future. That came in handy for my next trip, which was significantly longer.

Long Term Vacation Prep

September 2, 2017
I had known about the trip to Hawaii since I booked it in April 2017. So I had a lot of time and told myself I need to cut five pounds more than my target to be in a good place when I come back from my vacation. It turns out that, among other mistakes, hindsight also effectively identifies stress eating. The 5 lbs.-luxury I was hoping for, quickly went out the window when I looked at the scale. I didn't fully let myself think about it until a cookie and peanut butter meltdown – but it was a long trip with the added emotional layer of bringing my mom's ashes there. She'd always wanted to go, and I told her as soon as I could afford it, I would take her. It didn't turn out the way either of us planned, but I'm thankful I was able to go with my family.

The emotional aspect and being in a different country posed some challenges for sticking to a strict diet. By the vacation start I was a bit less than seven weeks from the competition, and by the time I got home I had five weeks and two days. At the eight-week mark, people start getting more serious about cutting, and by week four there are generally no cheat meals left. I left for Hawaii at 136.8lbs and 19.3% body fat and by some miracle came back at 137.7lbs and 19.9% body fat. OMG – so little TIME. I really wanted that 5lbs margin, but when I think about how much walking I did in Hawaii and how much I was able to see, maybe I wouldn't have if I had had those 5lbs to play with. Anyway, crunch time...

The tricks used in short-term stays don't pan out well when flights and a different country are involved, so you have to improvise. Knowing in advance that you will be away, you can plan two to three months in advance and change your diet to allow a five-pound weight cut when you get back. Then, when you're away you have that five pounds to play with. Basically, I suggest you do as I say, and not as I did, for your own sake! If you have a flight coming up, pack food for as much of the trip as you can. Also, while you wait for your plane, train, or bus, walk around as much as possible.

> *Being seated for hours on end or missing your workouts is not ideal, but keeping active while you wait lets you capitalize on your wait times.*

Being seated for hours on end or missing your workouts is not ideal, but keeping active while you wait lets you capitalize on your wait times. My husband, Patrick, and I had a flight delay on our way to Hawaii — during this time we made a workout video for anyone else who may be stranded and looking for something to do to pass the time. If you're stuck in a terminal or station somewhere, check my Naturopathically Fit YouTube Channel for many workout ideas.

Considering what I ate on some days of the trip, gaining only one pound was a HUGE win for me. I recall, on a road trip to Florida with three friends in university, I threw my food caution to the wind. As a result, I gained ten pounds in one week. BUT, for this trip to Hawaii, I made sure to book a hotel with a gym and also built physical activity into every day by walking everywhere, swimming and going on hikes. I highly recommend this because you can get up early, workout and then go enjoy your holiday or business trip. I went to the gym or did a hike eight of the ten days, including two travel days, and on the non-gym days I walked over 21,000 steps. I had cheat meals (explained later) on seven of the ten days, enjoying either a dessert or one meal, but the rest of the day was clean eating.

Without a step counter, the number of steps taken means absolutely nothing. To give you a point of reference, if I don't work out and just go to work at the clinic, I get 2,000 steps if I'm lucky, and this number is very common in people who have office jobs. If booking a hotel with a gym is not in your control, the next best thing is to increase your NEAT (non-exercise activity thermogenesis). This includes all activities you perform during your waking hours but excludes eating or exercise. For

> *...increase your NEAT (Non-Exercise Activity Thermogenesis). Take the stairs instead of the elevator, park farther away from the store, do yard work – anything that gets you moving more!*

example, taking the stairs instead of the elevator, parking farther away from the grocery store, or doing yard work, anything that gets you moving more!

When you travel you probably won't be carrying your food scale with you, so you go from measuring everything to eyeballing it. I ate a lot of hardboiled eggs, chicken and salad when I was away because I could easily keep track of calories in these things. Most places are pretty accommodating, but I was definitely the "Sally" from *When Harry Met Sally*. A couple of times at restaurants I would say, "Yes, I'd like the special chef salad, but please remove the fruit, nuts, cheese and dressing, but could you add chicken to this?" It was worth it though because I knew if I was eating on track for a couple of days, then I could eat pancakes for breakfast or manapua for a snack.

Keep in mind that if you are eating outside of your usual diet, be aware that the weight gain won't necessarily be all fat. Water retention can be huge, averaging anywhere from two to five pounds. For example, I lost four pounds in one week after returning from Hawaii but my body fat percentage did not change at all. So keep this in mind when you return from your trip. Trust that you'll stay close to being on-track if you put in the work.

> *If you're stuck in a terminal or station somewhere, check my* **Naturopathically Fit YouTube Channel** *for many workout ideas.*

Dr. Katelyn Butler-Birmingham

PART III: Training and Nutrition

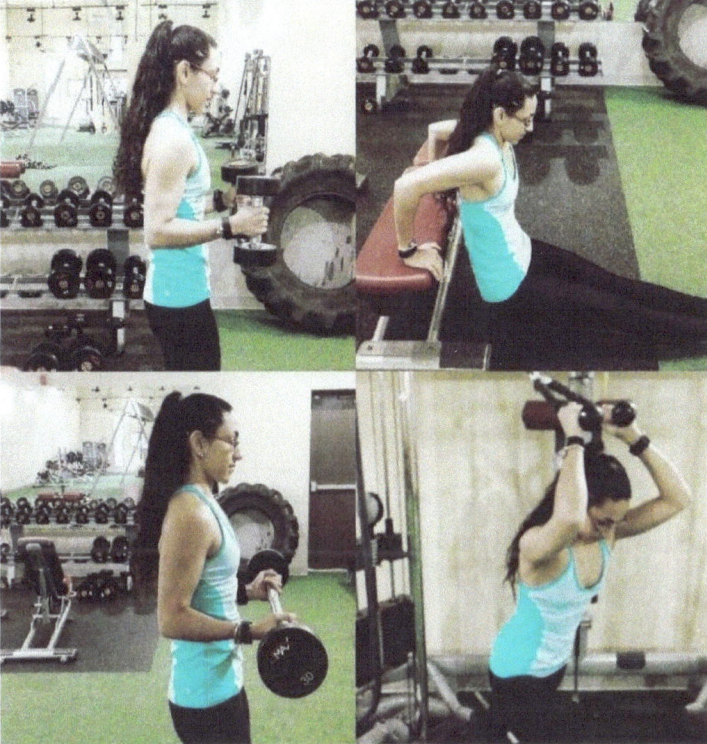

***This may look like hard work, but who knew it
actually would be the easy part?***

"Whenever I ask someone about their diet and they
say its 'good' or 'I eat healthy'– that's an immediate
red flag for me. No matter who you are, there is
always room for improvement."

– Dr. Katelyn Butler-Birmingham, ND

Individualized Training and Nutrition Plans

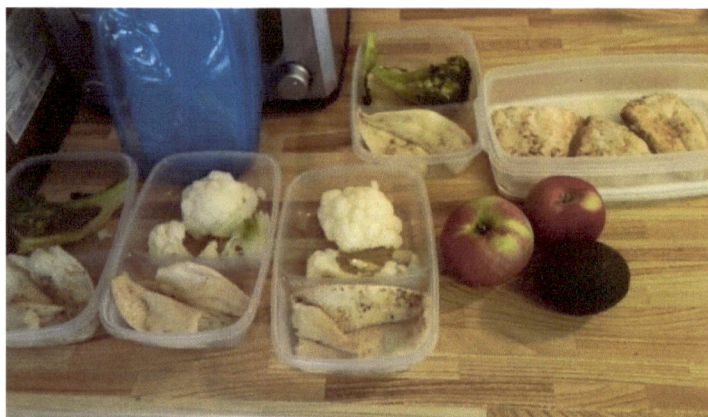

Tilapia, broccoli and cauliflower with an apple or avocado as a snack – very popular during crunch time

I wish I could put something down here that is concrete, that you could just read and follow and get the results you want. BUT, diet and exercise are VERY INDIVIDUAL. The words, *it depends*, come up a lot because people are vastly different in their body types, how their bodies respond to weight loss and what training style will give them the best results.

After having met several past competitors in Bikini and Figure, I've come to realize that when it comes to food, we had a similar reaction, and that essentially was feeling like you lost your mind at times. This happens to people when carbs are limited in an extreme way. The brain preferentially uses sugar to function, so it's no wonder that when carbs are scarce the brain freaks out.

Some people are affected by this more than others. I've had competitors tell me that when they are cutting weight their fiancée sleeps in another room. Another said she broke up and got back together with her boyfriend five times before the show. Others became hermits and avoided everyone and everything. The feelings that come up are anger, irritation, mood swings and fatigue. As I'm writing this, it sounds like prolonged and extreme PMS.

When you are in the strict cutting (weight loss) phase, two to four weeks out from the show, the core diet consists of lean proteins, such as chicken, turkey, tilapia, sole and basa, with dark green veggies like spinach, broccoli, green beans and asparagus. This is where most people start falling apart mentally. Food cravings are intense. Mood is not great, and fatigue really sets in. Having said that, if you plan things properly and lose weight slowly, the intense phase doesn't have to be so long.

People often ask me, "So what do you eat?" I tell them, basically lean proteins and veggies, mostly green ones. But, I quickly add that I would never recommend this diet to any of my patients. All the competitors I've met would not recommend the diet they eat to anyone else either. The reason for this is that it is not a realistic way to eat long term. The lack

85

of carbs, even if just from fruit, and the calorie restriction is not sustainable.

For a legitimate weight loss program to work and be maintained, you need to sit down, look at your current diet, start off with small changes, and make sure you include foods that you enjoy. Nothing should really be off limits, the frequency is what should decrease.

As soon as people start to feel limited, they want to rebel against the diet and end up sabotaging their efforts. So if, for example, I see that one of my patients needs help with their diet and they eat something sweet like chocolate, ice cream, cookies etc. after dinner, I first suggest that we switch that for a yogurt, or dark chocolate, or a piece of fruit, whichever they decide they are more likely to eat. Eventually you get them to eat the snack a bit earlier, then only four times a week, progressing until they stop their late night eating. Essentially you are looking to break habits gradually so that they aren't missed.

You can do this slow transition if you take a long time to train, but keep in mind your diet close to show time is not one you should stick to once the show is done. The ideal is to keep the base of your diet after the show and to slowly add in complex carbs like fruit, sweet potato, quinoa and brown rice.

When it comes to training programs, I have heard of several different styles. Some coaches develop training programs that are heavy on cardio — two hours per day, mixed with HIIT (high intensity interval training). Others focus more on weight-lifting and very little cardio. I did the latter, mostly because of my previous injuries, but also because I find weightlifting more fun. Your coach can vary this part of your routine, using something that realistically you will do. If you love cardio, that should be the bulk of your training. Keep in mind, however, the judges are looking at your shoulders and glutes, so you'll need exercises that work these areas. You may be someone who loses weight more quickly doing weights with a short 10- to 15-minute cardio session afterward. All plans need a trial run with your coach or personal trainer watching and assessing what works best.

We all have things in our diet we can't live without. Many coaches work around whatever item you refuse to give up. I didn't think there was anything I would be super sad to give up, but, turns out it's peanut butter. So, the second time around I built my meals around having peanut butter at some point in my day for the first month of training. Karen listed nut butter on three days in my week and that was better for me.

Other common indispensable foods I've heard of are coffee and cheese. The problem with coffee is it causes your body to lose more water. When training for something like this, you need to be drinking at least three litres per day, but if adding coffee, you need more than that. Some coaches say to drink an additional cup of water for every cup of coffee, black or green tea, however, it would take very special equipment to know exactly how much water that coffee or tea causes each person to lose, so this is just a guess.

On the bright side, once you have one show under your belt, you usually have more leeway with how much food you can eat because you know better how your body reacts. When Karen sent me a new meal plan for August, two months prior to the second show, I was excited to see that I had more meals listed and a greater variety.

What if you are **allergic** to some mainstays in the diet? Almonds and walnuts are all the rage right now, but I can't have them. With people who can't eat the usual stuff or just don't like it at all, you need to be creative. The required amounts of protein, carbo-hydrate and fat need to be calculated based on your height and weight and adjusted as you lose weight. However, below is a list of common foods used in the competition diet.

Protein makes up the majority of your diet. Most coaches use 1-1.8 grams of protein per kilogram of body weight to calculate your needs, then build the diet around that. Protein is very important because it is the foundation for building bigger, stronger muscles. Without adequate protein, muscles are broken down by the body.

Food list:

Veggies – Green beans, asparagus, broccoli, spinach,
   rapini, kale
Lean Proteins – Chicken, turkey, fish
Complex Carbs – Blueberries, sweet potato, brown
   rice, brown rice cakes, quinoa
Healthy Fats – Avocado, coconut oil, olive oil
Nuts - Almonds, walnuts, pistachios
Condiments – Nut butters (except peanut butter),
   mustard, sriracha, salsa, hummus

Expectations from this diet:

Water weight loss
Fat loss
Hunger!

I mentioned the food scale before; whatever you do,
DO NOT try to eyeball a portion size. It will not work
out. Our eyes or stomachs often tell us, "Ah, just a bit
more," and unfortunately those extra bits add up.
Also, make sure to know which foods are measured
raw vs. cooked. I learned the hard way that quinoa,
rice, pasta and sweet potato are measured cooked.
Lean proteins and veggies are measured raw. Make
sure to cover your scale or use a plate to measure
your chicken, turkey, fish, etc.

Most common types of exercise:

Weight training – for strength and hypertrophy
   (making muscles bigger)

HIIT – circuit style full body workout with weights or split training or cardio

Cardio – intervals or fast pace on the treadmill, stepper or bike

Expectations from the workouts:

Define and build muscle groups
Burn fat as fuel

Once you are limited to one or less cheat meal per week, you start to realize which foods have merit and which ones you thought were good but actually aren't worth wasting your precious calories on. Also recommended, is working out after a cheat meal or the next morning in a fasted state, to ensure you are using the carbs (fuel) you ingested. If for some reason you fall off the wagon, the body is pretty forgiving. If you have two cheat meals in a row, you are usually only up in water weight, but aim to be back on track by Day Three, because that's when you start regaining fat mass.

The cheat meal is there for a few reasons. Probably the most notable one is to curb cravings. Having a cheat meal at the end of the week gives you that light at the end of the tunnel. I do recommend eating it on Sunday night. I experimented with weekend breakfast and lunch, but I found it really tough to eat that cheat meal and then behave for the rest of the day. The calorie depletion during the week is like the buffer for the cheat meal that you have, so you can still lose weight, despite eating whatever you want for that meal.

Most people carb load for their cheat meal; this serves as a pump-up for the muscles. The further into the cut phase you get, especially if you're doing one month without any cheat meals, you notice that the muscles almost look flat, and the day after the cheat meal it literally looks like they've been inflated. This is the job of the final cheat meal. After being so carb depleted, the meal the day before the show is supposed to build

If, during your cheat meals, there is a time you overeat to the point that you are so full you are uncomfortable, I suggest you write it down in detail. Later, when you think you might like just a little bit more, or one more favourite item, read your note about how terrible you felt and it is easier to say no.

you up before you compete. The meal usually consists of steak, veggies and cheesecake; others do bacon, eggs and pancakes. Both ultimately give the same results. But, if done slowly and well planned, you won't have to go a whole month without a cheat meal, maybe two weeks at most. Make this process as individualized as possible so you are at your best.

February 2, 2017
Karen, Nathan, Marcin, Nathan's friend, and I all went to a specialty hamburger restaurant. I'll never go there again. My burger didn't even come with lettuce and tomato but it did come with a hair. Nope.

Everyone else loved their food but I'm officially done with there. Then the workout after sucked. I felt full and meat sweaty. Plus, I lost some weight on the leg machines so that's not good. Long story short, this weekend I'm eating a large Skor Blizzard after my workout! Mmm. Can't wait!

The second time around I didn't go crazy with cheat meals, at first. It was hard to predict what the next couple of months would bring, especially with vacation time in the mix. If, during your cheat meals, there is a time you overeat to the point of being so full you are uncomfortable, I suggest you write it down in detail. One of my good friends uses this trick, then when she thinks about eating just one more of her favorite items, she looks at her note about how terrible she felt after overeating. This is a great tactic, but you must commit to stopping what you're doing and going to read your notes for this to work.

Another option is to eat mindfully: taking in the cheat meal moment, truly tasting all the flavours, chewing your food, taking in the smells, texture and presentation. Numerous times, I made the mistake of not doing that and cheated myself out of the full experience – pun intended. When you savour every bit of your cheat meal, your body acknowledges you've eaten, you likely feel full before you gorge yourself and you truly feel like you've enjoyed your meal and busted your cravings for the week.

March 13, 2017
Before I kid myself - let me just say being overfull is way worse than feeling hungry. I had my cheat meal yesterday and it was a binge eat to the max. At least I'd learned my lesson and saved it until Sunday dinner. Being good all weekend is much easier when the cheat meal is Sunday...it was a feeding frenzy. I felt joy while eating. Complete joy. But after reflecting on the situation, I was so happy to be eating whatever I wanted that while stuffing my face with one thing I'd sample the next and keep thinking MMM! What's next? I did not get the full effect of the food right in front of me...How the hell did I fit in all that food? Sheer will. Then I proceeded to be extremely full the entire night with shortness of breath, couldn't find a comfortable position, night sweats, waking up thirsty, awake numerous times, unable to get back to sleep, and vivid dreams...

I wrote earlier about how prolonged stress on the body can lead to chronically elevated cortisol levels and that this can have a negative impact on the immune system. I bring this up again in the nutrition section because people tend to go for carbs at their cheat meals. As noted in my Instagram @naturopathicallyfit, I tended toward cookies, crackers, bread, muffins and chocolate. Logically, I know better, but it's different when you are in the moment.

Not big news, but remember bacteria feeds off sugar. If your immune system is lowered because of your intense workouts, having cake could set yourself up for a cold to sweep in. I know, personally, after a cheat meal I often wake up with a sore throat. So, I try to nip it in the bud with Vitamin C, lots of water and going to bed early.

Even with an extensive nutrition and fitness background, I strongly suggest having a personal trainer and/or coach who has experience in the fitness competition world. Having an objective eye to help you, takes the mental stress of finding tweaks for yourself out of the equation. You can get just the meal plan and plow through. Having them take progress photos and help you modify your workouts to maximize a certain muscle group is key. It is very hard to scrutinize your own body, even when using photos.

Recently, I was teaching a Healthy Eating and Weight Loss course and four of us in the group had competed in either Figure or Bikini categories. We showed each other photos and said things like, *oh I wish this was smaller or bigger, this isn't the best picture because . . .* We are our own toughest critics, so have someone else take a realistic look at what needs improvement.

> *We are our own toughest critics, so have someone else take a realistic look at what needs improvement.*

The experience from having a fitness background comes in handy when you need to improvise at the gym because the machine you want is taken, or you have an injury that is preventing you from doing certain movements. Also, when working out on your own and something doesn't feel quite right, you can modify the move or see flaws in your technique. Additionally, if you see you need to work more on a particular muscle group that is not part of your routine at that time, you can add it to your routine. For example, for the second show I wanted bigger glutes, more defined shoulders and abs, so when I had extra time I added them to the end of my workout.

Diet Tips and Tricks

"Always think positive. Keep talking to yourself. It is a mental game. You have to tell yourself that you can do it. See yourself on stage. When you step out there you want to know you did your best."

– Saadiya Ghanem, Personal Trainer,
Past Bikini Champion

When calories are so limited, and your goals so focused, tricks with food help you meet those goals without resorting to chemical supplements. Also, anything that makes food more palatable or keeps the hunger pangs at bay with that sense of having eaten, is very welcome.

Cinnamon – I learned about cinnamon in nutrition class at Naturopathic school. It was touted to improve insulin resistance with one teaspoon a day. I learned that, stored the information, and didn't think anything else of it until close to the show. About a month before the show, I told Karen, my coach, I didn't want to take diuretics or fat burners. She had a little panic, but then suggested I try cinnamon and cayenne.

I was a little skeptical at first, but the day I tried the cinnamon was a game changer. I mixed it in with my protein powder, Karbolyn, and water. I felt more energetic and less hungry than I had been. I thought maybe it was just a fluke, so I tried it the next day, and the next, getting the same result. It seemed to work wonders for about two to three weeks, then did not seem to work as well. I stopped using it all together, but if I had tried taking a break from it and going back, it may have worked again. Also it was getting closer and closer to show time where cravings take over, so the mental aspect could have been overriding the physical benefits.

Cayenne – is recommend by coaches because it is a very low-calorie spice you can add to just about anything. It is used to clear out the system and definitely does. If you can't handle spicy-hot things, this may not be the best option for you. It is often used in detoxes along with lemon juice because it increases circulation and gets the gastric juices flowing. It is also supposed to suppress appetite and boost metabolism.

I only used it for a month leading up to show time and was constantly hungry, but it can't hurt. For my second show I used it to spice at least one meal each day to see if long-term use made any difference. Looking back after completing my shows, I couldn't really pinpoint cayenne and say it made a huge difference, but it did make food more exciting.

Healthy fats – if you are at the major carb-cutting phase of your diet, your mood may be very low. I have tested healthy fats on myself to see if it can boost mood on its own. So far this seems to be the case. Cutting carbs and fat at the same time seems to be the problem. If you can add a healthy fat into your system, like a portion of butter, coconut oil, olive oil or avocado, this helps to stabilize the mood. My only caution is that healthy fats tend to have a higher calorie count, so keep this in mind.

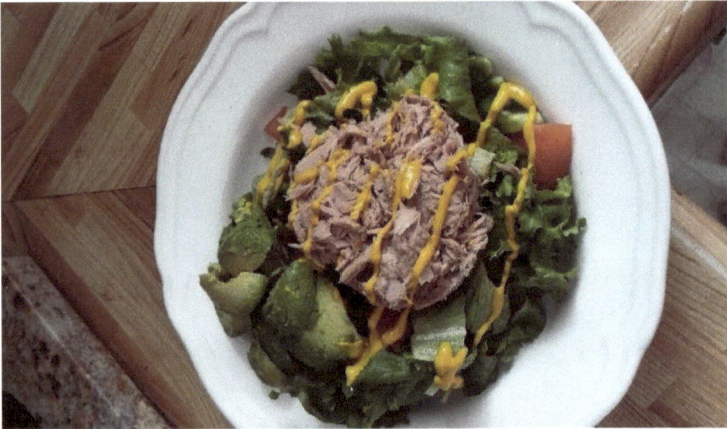

Who knew I'd be eating an avocado and tuna salad with mustard as dressing?!?

Condiments – There aren't many condiments that you can get away with when you're doing hard-core show preparation. BUT some have few calories and big taste to make up for it. For example:

1 Tbsp. Salsa=4 calories;
1 Tbsp. Mustard=10 calories;
1 Tbsp. Sriracha=10 calories;
1 Tbsp. Apple Cider Vinegar=3 calories.

I never thought I'd be using mustard as salad dressing, but you do what you gotta do!

Carbohydrates – Even in the serious carb-cutting phase, you can stand to have a small amount of carbs in your diet every three to four days. I notice if I'm doing three days straight of just lean proteins and veggies, I start to get cranky. So, I tried adding a banana. Work out the calories and your proteins so you are getting what you need, but notice what happens. My mood was better that whole day and I could go another few days riding on that high. Being grumpy all the time isn't worth it, so find out what the maximum number of days are that you can happily subsist on lean protein and veggies. Tell your coach and have them work additional carbs into your diet.

Gluten free – be cautious if something says gluten free. If you have celiac disease, or a wheat sensitivity this may be your only option for baked goods, but if you are not gluten sensitive, be cautious about choosing this option. Although gluten free is associated with eating healthy, that is not necessarily the case. Gluten helps bind things together, so when you remove this from baking, other things need to be added to help with consistency and it is typically sugar. Sugar can hide under many names like: dextrose, dextran, maltodextrin, maltose, galactose, glucose, sucrose, fructose and anything ending with syrup.

Another aid to reaching your goals is support from those around you, and replacing textures of favourite but disallowed foods. For example, if you know you have a gateway food (something that you eat knowing it throws you off your diet), make sure no one in your household buys it. If you feel you might fall off the wagon, have a tablespoon of nut butter. If

Dr. Katelyn Butler-Birmingham

you are still hungry, combine this with celery sticks. The celery sticks are filling, and if you're a chip person, the crunch may help you.

Nutrient Needs

Someone saw my progress photos on Instagram after my second show and asked me what I ate. They wanted to know portion size and all. I have no problem discussing food with people and often have a few curious about what I'm eating and why. It's fun to get into the nitty-gritty, but that's **my** nitty-gritty and may not be applicable whatsoever to the person asking me. If it were that simple, all competitors would have the same diet. There may be similarities, but nutrient needs are a huge factor for me when I provide patients with dietary advice and make recommendations on the diet they're currently following.

> *...many people are curious about what I'm eating and why. It's fun to get into the nitty-gritty, but that's **my** nitty-gritty and may not be applicable to that person whatsoever.*

Your nutrient status (i.e., assessing whether or not you are getting sufficient vitamins and minerals from your food) is based on several things. What you've eaten in the past, are currently eating, your age, your health, lifestyle, activity level, smoking, drugs, alcohol, medications and gender are just a few factors. The most common example is women taking birth control; most are unaware that it depletes vitamin B12. So, after taking their health history, I keep an eye out for it in their diet to see if it is being replenished and make note of any signs of deficiencies that may show up in their physical exam.

The person who asked me about my diet was a large male. So when I say my diet would not be applicable to most, it really wouldn't apply to him. Each meal plan is tailored to you individually. Proteins, fats, carbohydrates, hydration, calories and nutrient status are all taken into account and change based on your weight.

Female competitors get special treatment for their diet because there are variations that need to be made for menstrual cycle changes. These changes vary based on cycle length and flow (heavy versus light). This is no simple task, especially when trying to balance all of the factors above as well. As restrictive as the last month of dieting can be, you still want to ensure you're getting all the nutrients you need. This keeps your body functioning at its optimum during crunch time. One reason why starting slowly is important is so the last month does not have to be so extreme.

I attended a seminar by Dr. Ken Kinakin, DC, at the World Fitness Expo in Toronto in August 2017. His talk was on how to do a nutritional physical. When he started talking, I quickly realized he was using applied kinesiology.

Applied kinesiology has many uses, muscle testing being the main indicator for various things, including discerning nutritional or physical deficiencies. It takes an expert to determine the difference, but Dr. Kinakin talked about a few easy tests to determine a possible nutrient deficiency. As with any test, you have to take patient history, health status and symptom picture into account for the test to mean something. If nothing else, you have a couple of fun party tricks to show your friends. The iodine test and the Zinc Tally test are the most fun because the results are unmistakable.

Iodine test – A self-test done to estimate the body's iodine level using a liquid iodine solution on the skin and monitoring its disappearance over the course of a 24-hour period.

Materials needed:
- Betadine, 10% povidone-iodine antiseptic solution; can also use a 2% solution if needed, but be consistent from trial to trial.
- Q-tip® (cotton swab) or cotton ball

How to:
Use the dropper to soak the Q-tip® in the Betadine. Make a circle on your skin with the solution, using the inner aspect of your arm or forearm so you can see the results more clearly. Let dry completely. You can have clothes over the dried solution and you can shower with it on as well.

Interpreting Results:
According to Dr. Kinakin if the betadine fades within 24 hours, this indicates low iodine. With adequate levels, the spot will still be there 24 hours later.

Iodine Sufficiency	
Time	Iodine Deficiency
24+ hours	Sufficient
18-24 hours	Mild
12-17 hours	Moderate
11 hours or less	Severe

Zinc Tally Test – A self-test done to estimate the body's zinc level using a liquid zinc solution placed in the mouth for 10 seconds.

Materials needed:
- Zinc Tally (zinc sulphate); liquid form of zinc
- Teaspoon
- Small glass
- Stop watch

How to:
Put two teaspoons of the Zinc Tally in a small glass. Swish the solution in your mouth for at least 10 seconds. The liquid can either be swallowed or spit out after the test. The taste most people describe is metallic or strong, if they taste anything at all.

Interpreting Results:

Taste	Zinc Deficiency
Immediate	Sufficient
Delayed	Mild to moderate deficiency
None	Severe deficiency

The test that he talked about that really hit home for me was the iodine absorption screening test. He had Betadine with him so we could all try it if we wanted to. I put some betadine on my right bicep and waited to see what happened. Five hours later the iodine spot was almost completely gone.

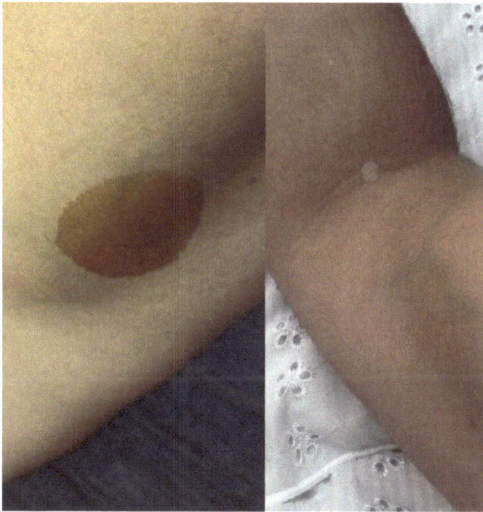

Iodine Test – Trial 1 – This is a photo of my right upper arm. In the photo on the left, I'm still at Dr. Kinakin's seminar. In the photo on the right, I'm home five hours later and the iodine spot is almost completely gone.

I wasn't overly surprised because in the past few months my hair had been shedding more than usual. I was also feeling cold all the time, and tired. Some other symptoms to watch for are low mood and trouble losing weight. The cold-all-the-time I could brush off because the more weight you lose, the more you feel the cold, and the fatigue I attributed to training and working long hours. But the hair loss was unmistakable. Every time I washed my hair I looked at this huge clump in my hand thinking if I continued at that pace my hair would be very thin in no time.

Clinical experience helps here because hair loss in clumps can be alopecia (if in patches), or from a fungal infection or autoimmune condition. These were easily ruled out based on overall hair loss and my symptoms. To be safe, I got my thyroid hormones tested to ensure I was in the normal range. I was; so I started taking an iodine supplement. I don't recommend doing this test on yourself unless you have a healthcare professional to monitor you. Messing with the thyroid can be very serious. By supplementing yourself with iodine, you can worsen an existing thyroid condition.

Not all supplements are created equal. Make sure to consult a Naturopath to ensure there won't be any interactions with your medications or other supplements you are taking. If you have your thyroid tested and the result is either hyperthyroidism (overactive) or hypothyroidism (underactive), you need medication to get this in balance. If your thyroid hormones are within normal range, but you still feel cold, tired, low mood, and hair falling out, this is a medical grey area – the presence of symptoms without any clinical signs. Naturopathic medicine thrives here because the symptoms can be managed although your test results would not qualify for prescription medication. It takes six to eight weeks of supplementation to have any stable effect on the thyroid gland.

October 16, 2017

So, it turns out getting liquid iodine isn't as simple as going to the drug store – they can order it for you, but Shoppers Drug Mart in London, Ontario, doesn't carry it. Luckily the second pharmacist recommended Shoppers Home Health Care. I thought they were one and the same, but they aren't! I only discovered this after thoroughly confusing myself and the pharmacist.

To conduct a retest of my iodine experiment I needed Betadine, which is a topical iodine solution. It needs to be at least 2% iodine. When I finally got to the right place, they were all out of the liquid form but had the wipes. Both work the same. Not many people order this, so I should have called ahead or I might have ended up on a wild goose chase.

The experiment is set for the next Saturday and I hope after eight weeks there will be some improvement. If the spot lasts longer than five hours, that means progress. I really didn't notice any changes up until this last week, after seven weeks of diligent supplementation. I've noticed a bit less hair loss in the past week or so.

Dr. Katelyn Butler-Birmingham

At the second trial, eight weeks after starting supplementation, the iodine spot was completely

> *You have to be careful with supplements.*

gone again by the five-hour mark. I had my thyroid tested again to ensure I was staying within the normal range. I reiterate, you must be careful with supplementation and monitor changes meticulously. Although the home testing with the liquid iodine visually appeared the same, the amount of my hair falling out decreased significantly from a clump the size of a golf ball to now being slightly bigger than a small marble. Likely, tracking my progress requires more trials, but that is reserved for another time.

Holidays and Special Occasions

"Time is simply how you live your life."

– Craig Sager

There is never a good time to do a show. There will always be holidays or special occasions some time during training. All I can suggest is to look in your planner, make note of when they are coming up and, if you can, schedule a cheat meal that day. Closer to the show, you may not have many left. So be picky when deciding in which meals you'll take part.

On a couple of occasions, I was the only one at the table not eating or having a completely different meal that I brought myself. All I can say is that preplanning is your best friend. Having snacks on hand or a prepacked meal when needed is essential. Honestly the only thing that saved me on a few occasions was knowing that the next day I had a cheat meal waiting for me.

The closer it got to competition time, the harder it was to watch people eat, even if they were eating something I would not normally choose. If you have to skip out on certain things, don't feel bad. Easter was four weeks from my first competition and I gave some SERIOUS thought to not going to our family dinner. The food cravings were getting bad at that point and I wasn't sure I would be able to handle watching people eat delicious food. I say watching because how food looks to me is what makes it appealing. For you it may be even just the smell. After some major back and forth, I did end up going. I ate before I went, which was a bad idea. I should have eaten there. I was okay during dinner, but not after dinner. When I went home and had no meals left, the cravings were insane.

So, test the waters with different methods. Pick something that works for you and go with it! The second time around I used many such tricks to get by when going to an event. One month out, I stopped going to things and dreaded going to the grocery store. The cravings were bad until about two weeks out when it seemed much easier. I could watch people eat and be okay with it because I could see the light at the end of the tunnel. It also helped that the day after the second show was Thanksgiving.

Calorie Counting

"The will to win is important, but the will to prepare is vital."

– Joe Paterno

Depending on how you feel about calorie counting, this may or may not be how you track your intake. Some people find it easier to use the macro breakdown. It tells you how many grams of each macromolecule (fat, carbohydrate and protein) you are allowed to have per day and you make the foods you choose fit into this format. Using an app like My Fitness Pal makes this easier for you. BUT, as you will soon learn, not all calories are created equal.

Zero calorie items will be very tempting, especially when you have few calories to work with. Don't be fooled by this. **Zero calorie is code for full of chemicals.** Some examples to watch for are: aspartame (Nutrasweet), sucralose (Splenda), saccharin (Sweet N' Low) and stevia (Pure Via), just to name a few. Stevia is one of the most popular sweeteners today because it is marketed as being safe because it is from a natural source – the stevia plant. It can safely be used if you consume the stevia plant as a whole, but not the refined white powder. What makes stevia like all the other sweeteners is that it has undergone a lot of processing to look the way it does and, like all artificial sweeteners, will impact blood sugar levels regardless of having no calories.

If we look at physiology for a moment, the pancreas releases insulin in response to glucose in the system. The pancreas is a very important organ that helps us with digestion as well as blood sugar regulation. Insulin is a hormone produced by the pancreas that pulls sugar into the body's cells so it can be used as fuel or stored for energy production at a later time. The body likes to be prepared though, so it doesn't wait for the sweet treat to get all the way down to the stomach before sending out insulin.

The body uses what is called a feed forward response. This means that as soon as something sweet touches the tongue, the brain interprets this and sends a message down to the pancreas saying, "Sugar is on the way; send out insulin to collect it." Of course the pancreas obliges and sends out insulin. Sugar is very quickly absorbed into the bloodstream and, under normal circumstances, floods the system so that insulin can match it and tell the cells to take up the sugar for use. If, however, you have ingested an artificial sweetener, the insulin will be hanging out in the blood stream wondering where the heck all the sugar is. With repeated use, the pancreas starts ignoring the messages to send out insulin because the others were false alarms. The body is pretty adaptable, so it can tolerate this boy-who-cried-wolf scenario for years, until one day you develop prediabetes or type II diabetes. Why? Because when you finally do eat something full of sugar, the pancreas won't send out enough insulin to help the sugar get into the cells. Instead, the sugar is left sitting in the blood stream. With time, this can damage blood vessels and lead to other problems like heart attack, stroke, kidney disease, and poor circulation causing sores and blindness. So when you reach for that natural Stevia, think twice about what it is really doing to your body.

Along that same vein, people often ask about brown sugar versus white sugar, or honey versus maple syrup. I say, if you're going to have sugar, do it and enjoy it. These examples all contain sugar that the body recognizes as such, so if enjoyed in moderation, you needn't worry about the health consequences of too much sugar. Ironically, the consequences are the same as when trying to trick the body with artificial sweeteners.

The health consequences of too much sugar are, ironically, the same consequences as when trying to trick the body with artificial sweeteners.

I chose to count calories so that I could just memorize the caloric value of a food and know if there was space for it in the day. I used My Fitness Pal until about two months out from the first competition. I realized looking at how few calories I was consuming actually made me feel hungrier than just weighing and packing food already calculated for protein content, carbs, fat and calories. As far as calories went, being ignorant of the numbers was much better the closer I got to the show. I then was able to put all my focus on fitting in all my meals.

Okay, I have five meals. How do I space these out so I don't eat within two or three hours of going to bed?

I had four to five meals a day for the first show, but I found it tough because it was like playing chess with my day. Every day is different for me with patient appointments and clients at the gym. You must find what works for you. Whatever you need to do to distract yourself from the hunger pangs, do it!

At those moments when you are looking in the cupboard, struggling to pick the lesser evil, it may help to think of the calorie content of a food in economic terms. What will this item cost me? Is it really worth it? The closer I got to my second show, the easier it got to say no to muffins, because the ones I like are 420 calories. This was a third of my calories for the day. So the choice was to eat one muffin and only have two meals for the rest of the day, or skip the muffin altogether.

Another way to think about it is to ask yourself if this food is helping to build you up or not. For example, will the food you're craving take up calories you need to get all your protein in for the day? I emphasize again – **Diet is Everything!** You can train six days a week for one to two hours a day like I was, but if you aren't eating what you're supposed to, the training will be for nothing.

For me, the diet was the toughest part. I love working out, so that was easy. Put the most effort into whichever area is the toughest for you. The safest bet is to choose whole foods, i.e., a diet that comes from fresh foods, nothing packaged at all, and supplement only the necessities specific to you. This ensures that you control at least one aspect of your chemical exposure.

Link Between Food, Mood and Health

"Let food be thy medicine and medicine be thy food."

- Hippocrates

When you decide to finally start preparing for a show, choose the best foods to fuel your body and mind. This is critical in maintaining health throughout this journey and allows you to maximize your workouts. I'm all about the Whole Foods Diet to accomplish this, but was even more convinced after reading an article, called "Bread and Other Edible Agents of Mental Disease," by Paola Bressan and Peter Kramer. This is one of the best articles I've read in a very long time. It has the perfect combination of research and layman's terms so it is easily understood. As I said before, I made mistakes during my fitness competition journey. The more you know, the more you can perform to your highest potential. A big part of that comes from your knowledge of food choices and their impact on your body.

Paola Bressan and Peter Kramer write:

> "...in all of us, bread (1) makes the gut more permeable and can thus encourage the migration of food particles to sites where they are not expected, prompting the immune system to attack both these particles and brain-relevant substances that

resemble them, and (2) releases opioid-like compounds, capable of causing mental derangement if they make it to the brain. A grain-free diet, although difficult to maintain (especially for those that need it the most), could improve the mental health of many and be a complete cure for others."

Salient points of the article:

- One in three people are negatively affected by wheat without having Celiac disease.
- One in six people have Celiac disease and have no idea.
- Stress can cause intestinal inflammation.
- You can suddenly become gluten sensitive in adulthood.
- Intestinal inflammation can make it easier for bacteria, toxins, and undigested pieces of food to get into your bloodstream.
- Gluten is contained in foods, such as bread, cake, pasta, pizza, beer, and is used as a binding agent in many products – even candy.
- An unhealthy gut is associated with: arthritis, asthma, type 1 diabetes, and multiple sclerosis.
- These effects are also seen with milk, rice, and corn.

When I was at Naturopathic College, we talked a lot about nutrition and its impact on health. It was not new information when I learned it, but we talked a lot about how changing the diet of children diagnosed with ADD, ADHD and autism spectrum disorders to one that is gluten- and dairy-free along with some tailored supplementation, could make as much as or more than a 50% difference in their behaviour, in as little as three to four weeks. This is huge because this is where the link between food and behaviour really starts to shine. The article mentioned above is a must-read. It applies to both children and seemingly healthy adults.

Whenever I'm going over food sensitivity with people, I tell them to pay attention to the obvious symptoms like constipation, diarrhea or acid reflux, but also subtle indicators like headache, trouble sleeping, low mood and mind fog.

Another good reason to stay away from the above listed foods is that they won't serve you while you are preparing for your show. The calorie-to-nutritional-value ratio is very low. I encourage you to read this article and review their references. Your food choices will serve you much better after doing so.

In addition to wheat, rice, corn and milk, sugar is another substance that greatly impacts us. You crave it like never before on some days, but keep in mind it may not be worth the calories or body effect. Sugar plays a huge role in gut inflammation, suppressing the immune system and blood sugar highs and lows. I tell patients to stay away from dairy and sugar when they are sick. Based on the article, adding wheat to that list would be a good idea, because sugar lowers your immune system's ability to fight off viruses or bacteria that have gotten into your system, and bacteria thrive on sugar.

If you have a cold, which is typically caused by a virus, and your immune system is busy fighting that, then you ingest sugar, any small amount of bad bacteria you may have picked up along the way can feed off of the sugar and start to overgrow because your immune system is busy fighting off the virus. Once your system recognizes it is under a dual attack, its defenses are divided. This makes a simple cold more powerful and it takes you longer to get better. Like our cells, bacteria pull in sugar to get energy and multiply. This can tip a tickle in your throat into a full-fledged cold.

Despite what sugar can do to our immune system, we still need it in our diet – but as a complex sugar, like in fruit or veggies. If you're a person who gets headaches, feels dizzy, lightheaded, nauseous or grumpy without food, you know what a sugar low feels like. The ideal is to maintain a fairly consistent blood sugar level throughout the day, so that you avoid the highs and lows of a sugar rush and then crash.

This becomes even more important when you're training because the fuel you put in your body needs to make up for all the hard work you're doing at the gym. In addition, if you haven't had anything to eat, you are more likely to binge on something you shouldn't. Also, the consistently low-carb aspect of the meal plan teaches your body to use fat as fuel. I didn't have that for my first show, so I was getting pretty tired by the last week.

The second time around, my body was much more responsive to the lack of carbs and I was more energized because fat was being used as a fuel source. That happens with prolonged training. However, as the preferred energy source of the brain, you can't discount sugar or glucose altogether, but when you are cutting, it is important to find your optimal carb intake so you can still be functional and have the energy to get through your day.

Let's switch gears here to shed some light on what physical activity, either too much or too little, can do to the body and how it impacts health.

During training, you are more susceptible to colds and flus because while you're working out, your body is producing cortisol, as talked about in Part II. Known as "the stress hormone", it is the go-to hormone consistently released whether the stressor is good or bad. Increased exercise means increased stress on the body, which means multiple and longer exposures to cortisol. When there is too much of it in your body, your immune system lowers so you are more susceptible to picking up a bug.

Don't be alarmed by the numbers on the graph. They are more to illustrate the point that being sedentary and being excessively active can both lead to disease. Being sedentary is more associated with chronic disease, and vigorous activity with acute disease. The chronic illnesses associated with inactivity are heart disease, stroke and diabetes. Whereas the acute illnesses associated with high levels of physical activity are colds, flus and injuries.

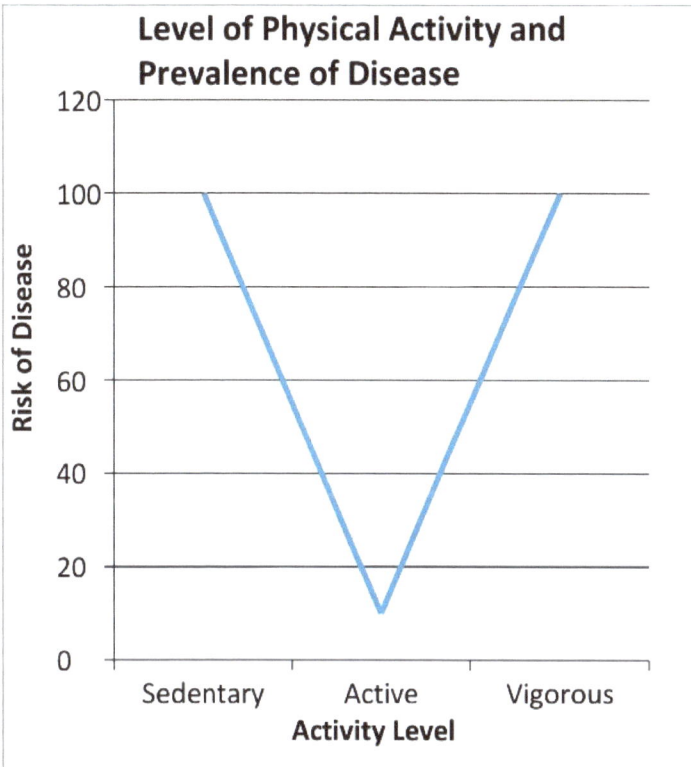

Level of Physical Activity and Prevalence of Disease

Y-axis: Risk of Disease (0, 20, 40, 60, 80, 100, 120)
X-axis: Activity Level (Sedentary, Active, Vigorous)

If you have ever run a marathon or know someone who has, you know that they are completely drained after the race and within a day or two often get a cold that knocks them out for a week or so. Also, sprains and strains happen, and in day-to-day life they're usually nothing to worry about because they heal in one to two weeks. In training mode, any little hurt can become a big problem and delay your training schedule. That is why self-care and stretching are the best things you can do for yourself.

For a happy medium, at least for before show prep and after a show, make activity part of your daily life without making it the sole focus of your day. The Canadian Heart and Stroke Foundation recommends adults should accumulate at least 150 minutes of moderate- to vigorous-intensity aerobic physical activity per week, in bouts of 10 minutes or more. To add to this,

Being sedentary and being excessively active can both lead to disease.

they recommend two full-body strength training days per week to maintain bone health.

On average, that means 30 minutes of moderate to vigorous activity five days a week. Several activities are classified as requiring moderate effort, such as a brisk walk, biking, raking leaves, swimming, dancing and water aerobics. Aerobics, basketball, fast swimming, fast dancing, hockey, and jogging are some vigorous effort activities. So if, for example, you choose one of the moderate to vigorous activities to do almost every day, you will be well on your way to health and fitness.

Imagine that you are extremely high on the vigorous activity side of things for a few months and your immune system is lowered due to cortisol and life stress, then you add in a cheat meal full of wheat and sugar, and you've got yourself the perfect setting for a cold. I've done this to myself numerous times.

Luckily, I had a great team of healthcare professionals to keep me going, but I recall many Sunday cheat meals with muffins, pie and you name it, then Monday morning I'd feel a sore throat starting. I did better for the second show and didn't put myself through so many ups and downs, but if you are a person who is already susceptible to colds, flu, and bronchitis, I really recommend doing your best to steer clear of this immune battle and focus on being your best self for when you step on stage.

Drying Out Phase

"Basically prepare yourself to camp out in your washroom. You will have to pee so much you may as well sit in there and make yourself comfortable."
— Anonymous Figure Competitor

Don't even think about this while you are prepping. Just worry about it when the time comes. BUT, do keep in mind that depending on what your job is, it may not be practical to do this for an extended amount of time. The length of the drying out phase will depend on how you look leading up to your show. The goal is to water load, then water and salt load, then deplete water and salt altogether, so that you look *tight* for the show.

When you have completed your month without a cheat meal – again, give or take based on how you look – the drying out phase sheds that extra two to three pounds of water weight. Because I did not use diuretics, Karen, my trainer, tried a longer drying out phase for me. I already had my water intake up to three litres per day on a regular basis, but for the water-loading phase I was consuming four litres per day and two pinches of salt on three meals for six days.

Keep in mind the water-loading phase can have you drinking as much as six litres per day. Then two days before the show it was down to two litres per day.

Then only one litre for the day before the show, and none after 6 pm. The day of the show, you get 500 ml for the entire day. Taking only small sips, you can make it last and maintain that tight look.

A little extra edge came from dry red wine. Karen had me drinking six ounces on the Thursday and eight ounces on the Friday before the show. I had to choke it down because to me it tastes terrible, but you may enjoy this part more than me. There are definitely no alcoholic beverages on the menu for a month or more prior to the show. Dry red wine contains tannins that act as a diuretic. I imagine black tea or coffee would have the same effect, but you may not be able to handle caffeine that late at night. Even if you could drink caffeine before bed previously, I don't recommend doing it the night before the show. After eating a very clean diet, caffeine, and alcohol too for that matter, hit you much harder. Generally, you have the wine after the competitors' meeting and then try to get some sleep.

I mentioned before that I found out about the posing changes the night before the show. The changes had been in place since last summer, but to me it was brand new. So, posing classes are a must! Keep on top of any changes so you are very prepared. I panicked at the meeting and then went home to practise. When I got there, I remembered I still had eight ounces of wine to drink. So there I am, drinking wine and trying to figure out this new posing. Not surprisingly, by the end of the glass the posing got worse, not better. I decided to call it a night before I twisted an ankle.

I only have a drink once or twice a year, if that. I don't really like the taste of wine, beer or liquor; the smell alone turns me off. So, because it took holding my nose to choke down the wine for the first show, I decided to opt out for the second.

> *After eating a very clean diet, caffeine, and alcohol too for that matter, hit you much harder.*

Wine is a diuretic, but also a vasodilator, which means it expands the blood vessels. So, for people with visible veins on their arms and legs, it really makes those pop, especially after the pre-show meal. I don't really have any visible veins to speak of, and wine is not my thing, so instead I had black tea – another type of diuretic. I finished 300 ml of tea around 4 pm the night of the show. If doing it again, I'd maximize the effect by doing the same amount the day before that as well.

It is good to experiment and learn what's best for you. Black tea is a very effective diuretic, so much so that my mouth was pretty dry by the following day. I didn't experience that with the wine. I'm happy with the results and definitely recommend tea as a substitute. It is effective, and it is low calorie. One cup of black tea is two calories, versus one cup of wine, which is 200 calories.

If you are looking very lean, you won't have to worry about the impact the final meal before the show has on your physique's appearance, but if you aren't as tight as you'd like, skip the wine and substitute black tea.

Dr. Katelyn Butler-Birmingham

PART IV:The Next Show

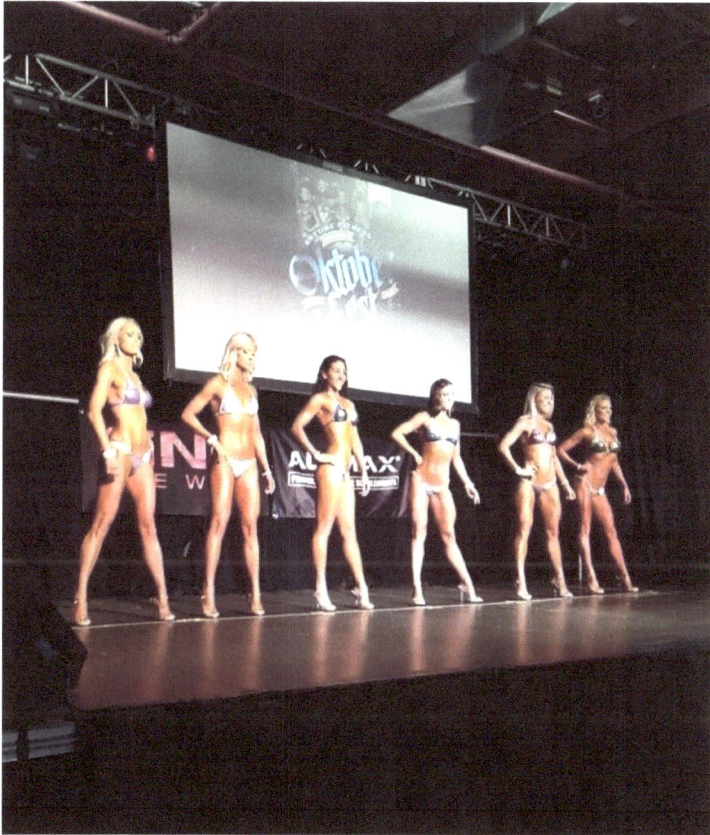

Oktoberfest KWOSHOW 2017

"If you aren't going to go all the way, why go at all?"
- Joe Namath

Oktoberfest: KWOSHOW 2017

September 13, 2017
Did I say Round 2 was easier? Hmm. Well, a lot is easier, like the muscles are there and you know what you have to do, but doing it is another whole story. I'd like to blame Dad for having muffins, pie and cookies in the house but, honestly, I could just choose to not eat them. Some days I don't even see them there, but this past weekend it was all I thought about. It's like I'm jonesing, literally. I keep getting the same thought about eating the food over and over; I feel twitchy, itchy, can't focus. And, if I eat it, then comes the guilt. Still can't believe how this feeling can overpower everything – logic and all. Today is the first good day of the week and the only difference is that I left home early and won't be back until 7:30 pm tonight. Being busy is key!

September 22, 2017
The struggle is real right now; the back and forth with food and wondering if I can hold out for these 2 weeks. It's just 2 weeks right? Why does it feel so hard right now? I want to eat that chocolate, and I can't even look at the muffins for fear of what might happen. I'd hoped my body would be better than it was last show, and I am stronger, but body-fat percentage says I'm bigger. I just want to get the show over with; yet I'm not mentally ready for it. With everything going on, I feel distracted and unfocused. Like, I'm so far from ready, it's not even funny. Sunday is the start of show meal prep but I'm

not ready. I'm freaking out and I got a sore throat midday Thursday so didn't want to push it. Went to bed early and didn't work out today. Will go on a hike tomorrow, but no workout. I need to rest and yet I feel this is when I should push – but the doctor in me says take your own advice and don't work out when you're sick. So, for now the plan is to get back into it on Monday – take the weekend to recoup physically, and mentally, I hope.

September 25, 2017

After the morning show at the Stephanie Worsfold Classic, I said I wouldn't do another show. But then, after all was said and done, I loved it and was already looking for another one for the same year. I don't know if it's crunch time talking or not, but I think this will be my last show for a while – maybe I'll try again in the Master's category when I'm 35. I'm definitely feeling how tough this is on my body. I took the weekend off and just walked, then started back today. Wow! I was moving at a snail's pace and the weights felt like boulders. Realistically, I should have taken another day off. I'm going to walk tomorrow and see how I feel. I'm in need of a good night's sleep too. So, I'm popping vitamin C tablets like the candy I wish they were, and hoping to feel better tomorrow.

Looking back and reading what I wrote is strange because I barely remember the time before the show. For the Oktoberfest competition itself, I could recount the entire day as a play-by-play, but I would have totally forgotten about having a cold. Clearly, this is another indicator the only thing that matters is that moment on stage for which you work so hard.

The second show was the 7th Natural OPA Oktoberfest. Overall, it was a great show. I'm not sure how it has been in the past. A smaller show, they made it more personalized by having us fill out cue cards with anything we wanted to have read as we came onstage individually for the night show. Many people wrote a shout out to their Mom, friends, or listed all the foods they wanted to eat after the show. It was really nice to hear the blurbs. They made the night show longer, but it was worth it. I have a video clip of my night show entrance on my Facebook page. The summary I chose to go with is that I'm a Naturopathic Doctor who teaches people about healthy eating and lifestyle by being the example. I knew by the second show that this book would exist, so saved the shout outs for here and let the business person in me take over for the show.

I'm not sure why, but the backstage areas at the two shows that I did, were very small, with little room to pump up. The athletes for the KWOSHOW were in a tent outside the venue. I thought they were joking. Luckily, the weather held for the most part that day, because there was a gap between the tent roof and the doors to enter the venue. Once again the volunteers for the event were amazing. They informed people of where to go, and lined us up perfectly to go on stage. It was a smaller venue, so for the morning and night shows there was standing room only by mid-show. The doors opened 45 minutes before the show started, so you might want to advise your guests to arrive at that time, or shortly thereafter, to ensure a good seat.

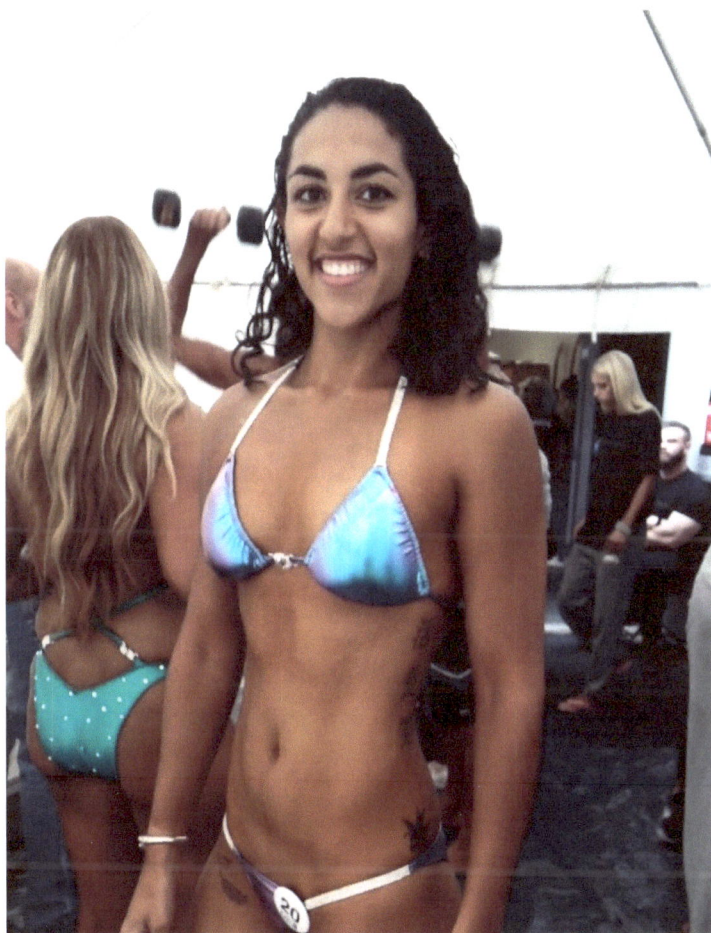

Inside the famous tent

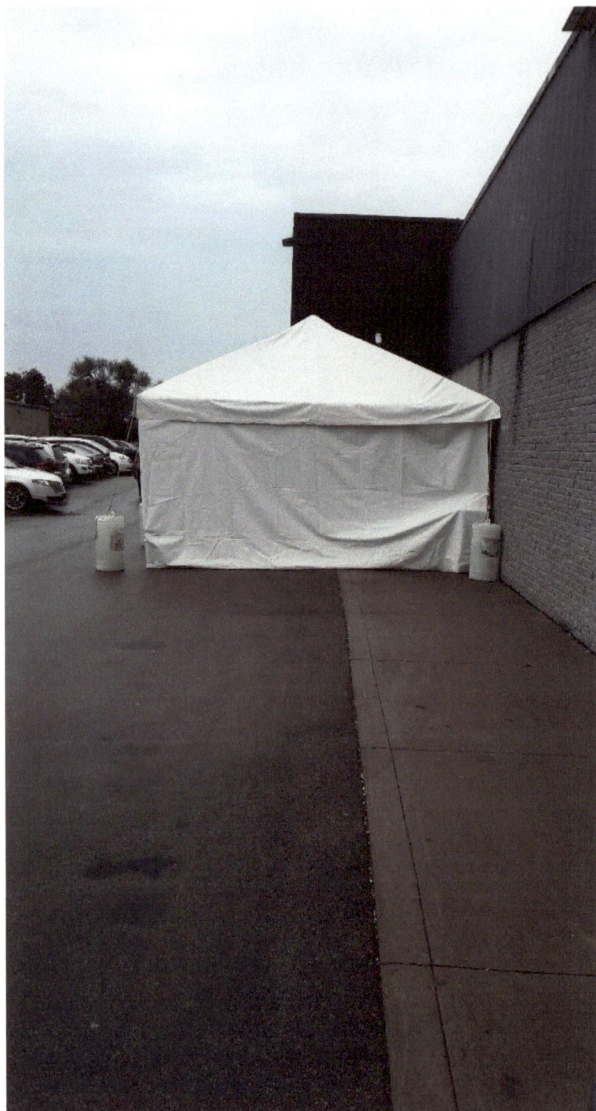

The famous tent from the outside

Comparing the Shows

	Stephanie Worsfold	Oktoberfest KWOSHOW
City	London, ON	Kitchener, ON
Venue	London Music Hall	Maxwells
Organizer	Stephanie Worsfold	Melissa Shadd
Head Judge	Rudy Jambrosic	Rudy Jambrosic
Show Times	10 am and 6 pm	9 am and 3 pm
Athlete Registration	$100 online, $125 at the athletes' meeting	$100 online or at the athletes' meeting
Ticket Cost	$25 for morning show, $40 for night show, $50 VIP pass, $100 for a coach's pass	$25 for morning show, $40 for night show, $80 for VIP (get seating in first 2 rows and access to morning and night shows), $90 for a coach's pass
Where to get the Tickets	Online, cash at the door	Healthy You Supplements in Kitchener, cash at the door
Accommodation	Home town	Delta Hotel $159/night
Stage Setup	Enter on stage right, exit on stage left	Enter and exit on stage right

Continued

	Stephanie Worsfold	Oktoberfest KWOSHOW
Night Show	2 of your favorite poses	3 of your favorite poses
Photos	Packages available from $90-120	Packages available from $90-120
Personalized	No	Yes
Spray Tan associated with event	Absolute Touch	Absolute Touch
Free Service	No	Bikini bite, free photos by Kitchener Muscle
Vendors	Many – lots of giveaways and samples	A bit less, but free samples and draws to win items
Volunteers	Excellent	Excellent
Backstage	1 long hallway with small open area at the exit steps	Covered Tent
Name lists	1	2
Total # of Competitors	Approx. 118	Approx. 79
# of Bikini Competitors	34	23

I really enjoyed both shows, but I loved the fact that the Kitchener show was done by 5:30 pm. Starting early and finishing early was great because I felt like we had the whole night to celebrate!

PART V: The Wrap Up

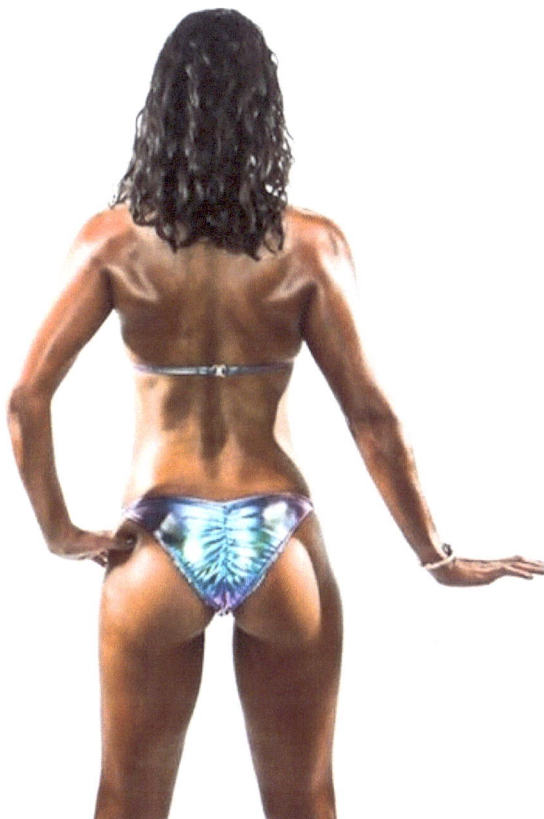

In Retrospect

"Strength doesn't come from what you can do. It comes from overcoming the things you once thought you couldn't."

– totalfitnessexperience.com

The Recovery

"Investing in a healthy lifestyle now, creates the greatest payoff."

> - Patrick Kangalee,
> Transport Economist

The first show is over. I finally made it. Most of us are so excited to relax and EAT after the show. Well, that and have a shower – with no shower after the spray tan and spray gloss applied twice that day it can feel very sticky! My coach told me to take it easy with the food re-introduction. I heard from other competitors that you can gain all your weight back within two weeks. Well when I heard that, I was shocked. How does that happen!? Now I know...

When I started my journey in December 2016, my starting weight was 136 pounds and I ended up at 123 pounds five months later for my first show. For my second show I started at 146 pounds and ended at 129 pounds three and a half months later. The yo-yo I did can be avoided.

The second time around, I allowed myself a week to eat what I wanted, while still eating what I needed to get my required protein. Although the numbers on the scale were not so different, I saw a big visual difference from when I started to train for the first show to being ready for the second. Despite being heavier for the second show, I was physically smaller.

Muscle is heavier than fat – that's not just a saying! Another reason NOT to live by the scale.

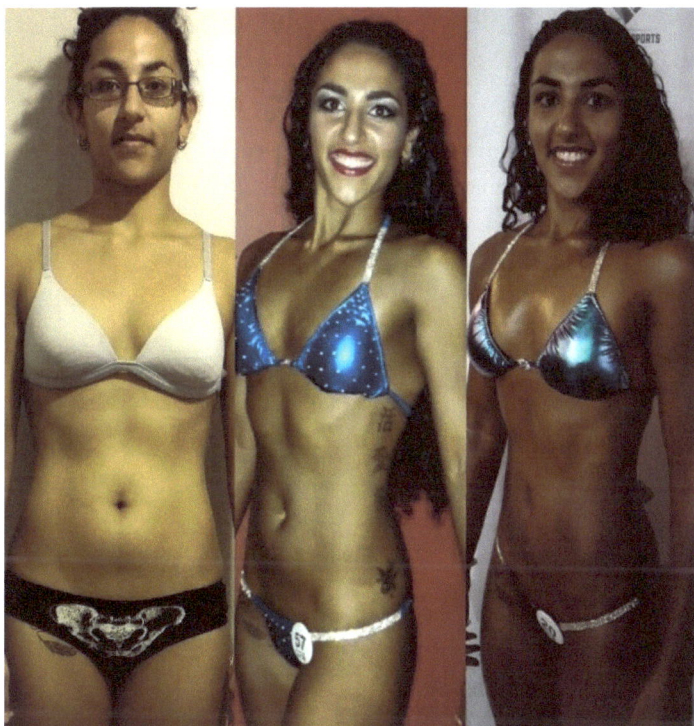

Start in December 2016, 1st show May 2017 and 2nd show October 2017

The first time around, I went food crazy. After the show I had pizza, cheesecake, cookies, M&Ms and hot chocolate. Unfortunately, it didn't stop there. I didn't even recognize myself when I was making food choices and that continued for the next month. So I definitely gained back all the weight I had lost, and even added ten pounds by the end of the food-crazy month. The first show was May 13th, 2017. The extreme food cravings started to subside around June 9th, 2017. I told myself I would start getting my diet together at the beginning of July 2017.

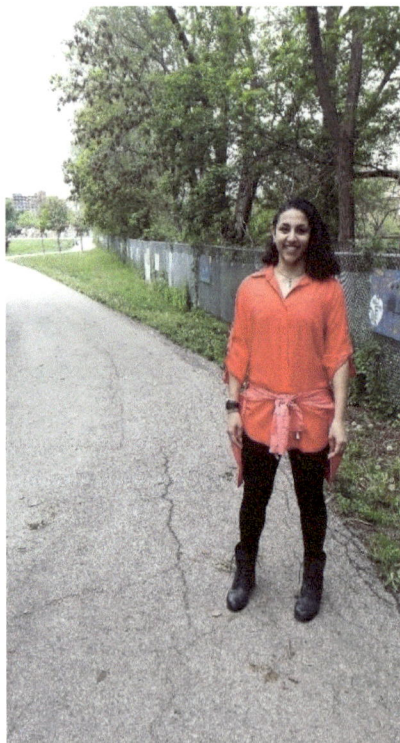

The drastic change from May 13th, 2017 to May 27, 2017 after going food crazy

Then started the slow process of making better choices. The week after Canada Day I was on the right path again and had already dropped five pounds in a week. It can be that fast – in either direction. In my practice I have seen someone gain nine pounds just by eating something they didn't have in their diet before. Water weight is sneaky like that. Then when they cut out wheat again, they dropped right back down a few days later. So I will take this opportunity to really drive home that diet is everything.

That month when I was going food crazy, I was still at the gym for an hour and a half six times a week, and on the off days walking for about two hours. I also challenged the staff at Martin Wellness to a month-long step challenge.

> *I was full and happy, but after hearing others' experiences, I realized that wasn't the norm.*

Melissa Martin, life coach *extraordinaire*, was my biggest competition and had me working VERY hard for the win. Even so, I still gained all that weight. Then, when I started making better choices, as I said, an easy five pounds came right off. Keep in mind that a healthy weight loss pace is one to two pounds per week. That is after the initial water weight drop that most people get after cutting out certain foods.

The night of my first show I was up until 2 a.m. posting pictures on Instagram, making photo layouts and looking for another show. So if you are considering doing another show, give yourself some time to get your bearings back. Unless, of course, you win the competition and qualify for the next level.

Often that is a week or a month later depending on timing.

Well, you have an idea how my recovery went after the first show. I ate all the foods I wanted and ballooned out. Yet, I was really happy at the time. I'm also happy that I worked out throughout the binge phase because once I was losing again I could see the muscle maturity and had hopes that I'd be bigger and stronger by the next show. Knowing what to expect from my body, I was able to fine tune things for the second show. I remember thinking I'd learned my lesson about the binge eating on junk food, but wondered if I'd feel completely different about it in October.

After being in a show you tend to meet others who have done the same. I had at least three people ask me how my recovery was going. I thought to myself, "What recovery?" I was full and happy. However, after hearing their experiences, I realized mine wasn't the norm.

> *The body you have at the show only lasts for one or two days.*

One woman told me that her body image was so bad after the competition she battled with intense bouts of depression for three months after the show. She got so used to her body looking one way, then after the show she felt fat and couldn't get used to how her body looked.

The body you have at the show only lasts for one or two days. I know I've said this before, but it really is a hard concept for people to understand, especially for those having the experience. The reason for that is you've gone through a lot during the difficult drying out phase. Then post-show, all you think about are your favourite foods and how quickly you can get them. After the drying out phase you are the tightest you will ever look and it is unrealistic to hold yourself

> *How different their experiences would have been if they only used food and water instead of fat burners and diuretics.*

to that standard. Eating so few calories and carbs is not sustainable over the long run, so you need to prepare yourself for the new norm after the show is done.

Another woman who was in the Figure category, as mentioned briefly before, told me that even years later, her body was not the same. She said that she got so small for the show using fat burners and diuretics that her body had not bounced back. She felt a stronger, shorter build was her norm, but going that small was too much and the look of her body had changed permanently. Hearing these stories, I thought to myself, "How different their experiences would have been if their coach had used only food and water to fuel them, instead of fat burners and diuretics."

Recovery Again

After the first show, I was thoroughly convinced that the weight regain can happen within a week, so after the second show I decided to do it differently. Deciding not to go food crazy and actually not going food crazy are two different things. I was not eating like the first time around, where I had cake, cookies, pie, Cheetos, etc., but it still wasn't great; bread made a vicious come back on my menu.

I felt more relaxed around food, no longer feeling like it would disappear if it wasn't devoured. I also had the added motivation of doing a group blood donation in November 2017. Having it close to the show was great because it helped remind me that people were counting on me to be at my best. Lives literally depend on it. That is a big responsibility. Even without that, I want to be a role model to my clients and patients. I can only expect clients to take my advice seriously, if I'm following it myself.

October 9, 2017
Patrick, Yaz and I were watching the show while the Physique guys were up there. Patrick is goofing around posing like them, flexing his muscles, and then got serious and was like, "You know, I want to try this, I could do this right?" But something made me think that when he said I, he was really saying we. Crap. I had already decided I didn't want to do any more shows for a long time, maybe not until I was in the Masters category, if then. But if he does

one, I could do one. It would be easier to do it with a partner. I said, "Okay, but not this year." The next day he's trying to eat healthy and then says he wants chips and buys some. So, ultimately, I suggested we do a photo shoot first. Let's just ease into it and see how it goes...

I'm happy to have another goal to work toward, having decided on the photo shoot. My goal was going to be to bench press my own body weight, but that one will have to wait. My best suggestion for a smooth recovery is to set another health goal right away to stay on track. Keep in mind that your body will be like a sponge. It will soak up all the carbs you put into it and try to hold on to them for dear life. So make it slow and steady until you're incorporating all the food groups you want.

Keep in mind that your body will be like a sponge. It will soak up all the carbs you put into it and try to hold on to them for dear life.

Surprises

"Life is 10% what happens to me and 90% of how I react to it."

– Charles Swindoll

Although I had past competitors give me tips about certain things, there were some surprises along the way. Some good, some strange and some in between.

I thought I had compassion for people with food addiction and weight loss struggles, but I don't think I fully *got it* until I was in it.

February 15, 2017
I finally understand the weight loss battle. I don't think you get it until you see the scale at a standstill, or worse yet – your weight has gone up despite feeling like you've been a rock star...The disappointment I felt when I saw my weight go up was crazy. I never thought a number would bother me so much, but clearly it bothered me for a whole two weeks. I'm actually dreading stepping on the scale this Friday morning. When you see the numbers stagnate – self-sabotage ensues. At least for me. I subconsciously was like, Fuck it! And started eating a bunch of peanut butter. Then felt guilty about it. I've never felt guilty about food ever! And I think about food all the time, even foods I usually don't like.

If this happens to you, have someone else keep your measurement records and not tell you what the values are. If your weight has stayed the same, or increased, there is something in your diet that needs tweaking.

Avoid doing a weigh-in until four to seven days after a cheat meal. I have seen people gain five to nine pounds in just water weight. This is nothing to worry about, but it can be awful to see on the scale.

I haven't had the chance to confer with any other past participants about this next one, but I noticed that the smaller I got, the more uncomfortable my bed became. I tend not to move much when I sleep, so having little padding on your body can make the springs seem like they are massive. I woke up every so often just to turn over. Also if you are a bit clumsy, you will quickly learn that running into things hurts significantly more than it did before. I went to sit down on the couch, just clipped the side of the armrest and hit my tailbone. I've done this before, so it was probably worse because of that, but it felt like I barely bumped it and it is still sensitive in certain positions four months later.

The last meal – as you get closer to your show, there is a light at the end of the tunnel. Almost as exciting as being in the show is the special meal you get the day or night before the show. The most common ones are steak and cheesecake or bacon, eggs and pancakes. The reason behind this is that you have done one month with no cheat meals, so you're very depleted and the muscles are looking flat. This one meal, then, gives you a little pump-up before the show, where you don't eat much of anything.

Some people can have the cheat meal for breakfast and then go back to eating what they should the rest of the day, but if this isn't you, I recommend eating the cheat meal for dinner. I packed my food and brought it to the competitors' meeting because I didn't want to be eating at 9 pm.

My meal was homemade steak, asparagus and cheesecake. I had a special cheesecake made for me that had an Oreo cookie base and peanut butter cheesecake, topped with chocolate and peanuts. Some people go to The Keg as they have this type of dish. BUT, if for some reason, you have fallen off the diet bandwagon and aren't looking as tight as you should the night before the show, you may be stuck eating chicken and spinach for your last meal before the show. Cracking down and focusing for that last month means you get to have a long awaited treat – a great last meal!

Hours of food videos – The last two weeks were tough. All I thought about in my spare time were all the foods I wanted to eat. I spent hours on Facebook looking at Goodful videos of cooking with healthy recipes. I would watch the dessert ones over and over and tell myself I was going to make them as soon as I could go back to eating normally. It has been almost three months since the first competition. Have I made a single dessert yet? No. I thought it was crazy for me to be obsessing over food videos, but I met another competitor who watched hours of The Food Network. I felt better knowing this. However, I hoped the second time around I could stick to reading motivational quotes or watching those types of videos. I actually used the time to find quotes for this book and talk to people who inspire me, which helped.

Clear skin – for many of us, adult acne IS a thing. We thought we left it behind in the teen years, but somehow it followed us to adulthood. Well, once you start taking care of yourself, especially cleaning up your diet, adult acne seems to fade away, until the cheat meal. I woke up the morning after with a breakout. Monday-Saturday my skin looked great.

Some people forget that skin is an organ; the largest organ of the body. It responds very quickly to changes in your environment whether they be external, like goose bumps in response to cold or sweating in response to heat, or internal, where what you eat becomes part of each and every cell in the body. The cleaner your diet, the fresher your skin.

Body odour – After hearing that there was absolutely no showering or wearing deodorant post-spray tan, I was concerned. I imagined all these people packed backstage with their anxiety sweat hanging in the air. Thankfully, I was wrong. I have worn an antiperspirant for a long time, not for lack of trying oils, making my own deodorant and the rock style ones. None of these seemed to work, but I figured if my skin was clearing up then my body overall must be doing the same. So I switched to a men's deodorant that doesn't stop you from sweating like ones with antiperspirant do. Lo and behold, it actually worked! I could do an intense workout and not have people dropping around me. That, and I could wear my clinic shirts all day, take them off and they would still smell fresh. This must have happened to everyone else, because no one smelled like much of anything other than spray tan. Don't get me wrong, people were still sweating. If you sweat a lot with a spray tan it shows. You see small lines where the sweat has run down your tan. This is where the touchups come in handy for you. Despite the sweating, there was still no smell to speak of.

Shrinking of the assets – Most women notice that if they lose weight, their bust and butt go with it. I often have people ask me, "How do I lose weight in my stomach area? Just my thighs? Just my love handles?" Well, unfortunately spot treatment does not exist with healthy weight loss. You will notice losses in the whole body. Where you see loss first or where you have stubborn areas is linked more to genetics than anything else.

Unfortunately, the breasts and bum shrink along with the rest of you. If you are small chested like me, it will be a slow loss of boob, with a transition to pecs, which in my mind looks nicer because they are well shaped and perky from the muscle definition. Also, don't be sad about your bum, it may be smaller, but it will be solid muscle which is pretty awesome!

Atmosphere at the show – A few people have asked me what it was like backstage. Was it catty or supportive? Some people were a bundle of nerves, some were quiet, but most people would smile as you walked by, help you if you were lost or fix your suit if it wasn't sitting right. While we were in line waiting to go on stage, most people chatted with the person in front of them, a couple of women called out saying good luck, let's have fun, etc. Everyone works so hard to be at the show. I think there is an automatic respect for the people around you because you know what it has taken to get there.

Gum – I haven't been an avid gum chewer since my high school days, but I can tell you I've tried at least 20 different brands since my first show. If you can get a good gum, with flavour that lasts, it is a good distraction when the hunger pangs are intense. The ones whose flavour didn't last for me are: Sour Patch Kids, Juicy Fruit (also the taste has changed since I had it last), most of the Trident gums except Spearmint and Excel Spearmint. The ones I liked best were Excel Winter Fresh or Polar Ice, Pur (If you are worried about aspartame they have pretty good chocolate, bubble gum and cinnamon flavours.), and last, but not least Dentyne Fire. During preparation for the first show I relied heavily on gum for the competition. The second time around, I used Werther's hard candy and Trident gum; ultimately very sparingly because one hard candy has 20 calories versus a piece of gum, which has five or less. It was helpful as a distraction, but you could also use flavoured toothpicks to keep your mouth busy and not worry about how many toothpicks you've gone through.

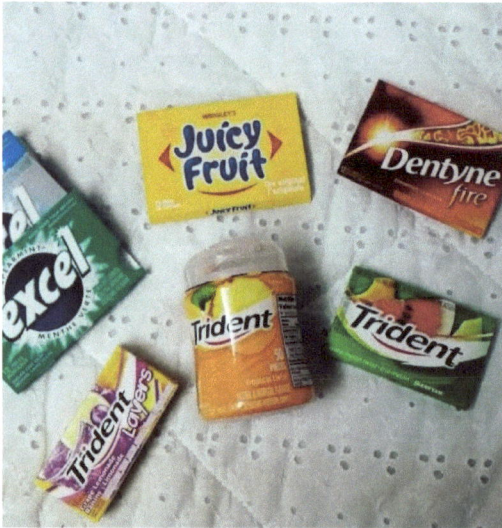

*For the first show I had a very impressive
gum collection to curb cravings*

Another surprise was looking back at how much my idea of meal planning has changed. Most people have a set idea of what breakfast, lunch and dinner should look like. In university, I used to think it was cereal for breakfast, eggs and sausage on the weekends, sandwich for lunch with yogurt and a granola bar, then dinner was some sort of meat with a salad. This slowly changed to having minimal grain products and the only dairy was milk in my tea. Once you decide to do the competition, let go of your idea of what breakfast, lunch, and dinner look like. At one point I was having tilapia and asparagus for breakfast and egg whites with spinach for dinner.

Even the smallest adjustment to meal timing can mean weight loss. I found that switching the meals around helped me look at food as fuel; on the good days that is. On the bad days, the food cravings were so intense I thought I'd lose my mind. I recall many times craving foods that I normally wouldn't touch. Yet somehow, all of a sudden these foods look amazing. For me, No Name chocolate chip cookies are hard and dry, but seeing them with my craving brain they looked like the softest, chewiest and most delicious cookies I'd ever seen! So if I could see food as fuel 100% of the time, it would really have limited the amount of time I spent thinking about junk food.

If it were possible for people to have no emotional, traditional or cultural connection to food, we'd all be better off. How often do people eat comfort food? Or need to have it because it's a tradition, eat it because they're bored, and the list goes on. If we only ate what we had to, when we were actually hungry it wouldn't be such a mental game to get competition ready. There are many intelligent species out there, but as far as I know, humans are the only ones who can put so much pleasure and guilt into food.

Physiological changes – If you have a fitness tracker I strongly recommend wearing it. If you don't have one, you can log the changes manually. I had a Fitbit HR and have since switched to the Alta. I had to replace the HR model and was on my fourth one in less than two years. Keep in mind I wear mine all the time except for showering, so I really get lots of use out of it. I recommend purchasing the additional insurance if you decide to buy this product because they are good at replacing them.

One of the things I like best about this product is the FitBit app on my phone. I like being able to have step challenges with friends and see their progress week-to-week, and I like the sleep and heart rate monitoring features. The neat thing about heart rate tracking is I was able to see my resting heart rate and how much effort it takes for a certain activity, and how that changed with training. Before I started training for my first show, my resting heart rate would fluctuate between 70-75 beats per minute. The average adult heart rate in a healthy range can be anywhere from 60-100 beats per minute. The closer it got to my show, the lower my heart rate was. (See Figure 1.) Two weeks from show-time it was between 46-49 beats per minute.

The body is so neat that way. The more trained it becomes, the more efficient the heart is at pumping blood around the body. Here are two of the many reasons for this. First, you're losing weight; one pound of fat takes thousands of tiny blood vessels (capillaries) to feed it. Once the fat cells shrink down, they don't need as much blood flow to keep them alive, so cutting down on the number of blood vessels means less work for the heart. Second, the heart slows down because as you get more fit, your heart gets more robust, too. It becomes more efficient at pumping, so with each beat, the heart pumps out more blood per squeeze. For example, if before starting to work out your resting stroke volume (amount of blood pumped out of the heart with each beat) was 70 ml/beat, after working out for a few months it goes up to 100 ml/beat. If your heart can pump out more blood per beat, it doesn't have to beat as frequently.

Figure 1: Comparison of Weight and Heart Rate

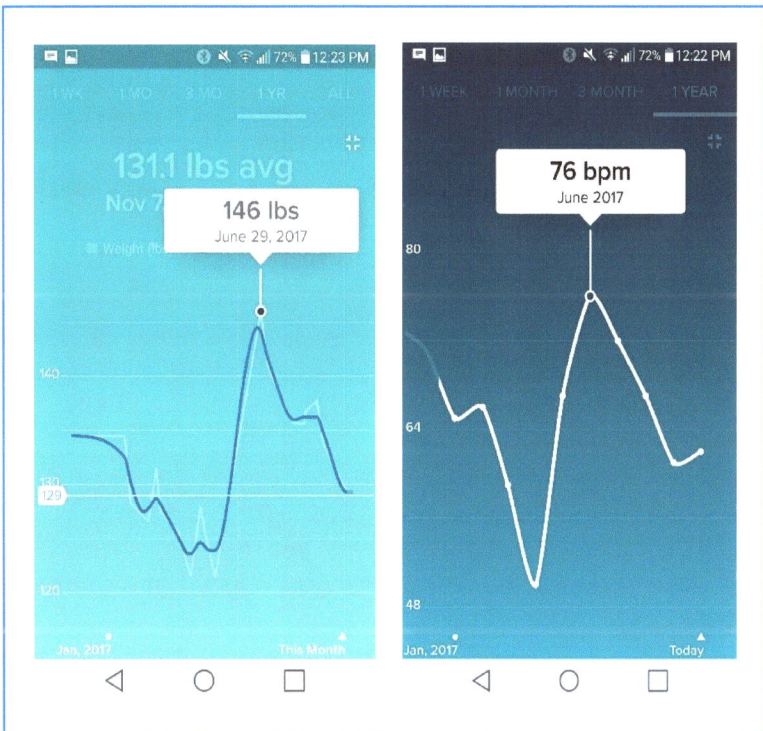

Dr. Katelyn Butler-Birmingham

The screen shots of my Fitbit app show the contrast of my weight going down and my heart rate following, then in June showing what happened to my heart rate when my weight skyrocketed.

If you don't have a fitness tracker with a heart-rate feature, you can keep tabs on this manually. To check your own resting heart rate, have a timer with a second hand ready. Sit comfortably and quietly for 5-10 minutes. Hold out your hand (right or left, it doesn't matter which one) palm up as if holding a bowl of soup. With your other hand, take the index and middle fingers held together and place them just below the wrist crease (line where your palm meets the wrist) on the thumb side of your wrist. This is called your radial pulse. If you make a mistake and are on the pinky side of your wrist, you may also be able to feel the ulnar pulse, but it tends to be fainter and not as easily found.

Once you find the pulse, look at the timer and count how many beats you feel in 30 seconds. Then, multiply this number by two to get the number of beats in 60 seconds. For example, if you count 35 beats in 30 seconds, you get 35 X 2 = 70. This means your resting heart rate is 70 beats per minute. Check this once a week as you train and see what your results are.

What I Learned

"If there's one thing I've learned, it's never to hide who you are. Be yourself. That's how you truly connect with others."

– Jeremie McClean,
Isagenix Associate

Food is not just food. It can be an aspect of comfort, boredom, joy, addiction, tradition and so much more. This is why humans don't only view it as fuel, even if, as I mentioned before, it would be better if we did. And, when there is a shortage or an excess of it in your life, it begins to take on new meanings. I'm no stranger to secret eating and now I've had a glimpse into food addiction. Some clients at the gym comment that I

> *There are many thin people who have terrible diets, and overweight people who eat well. You never know what someone's relationship to food is, until they tell you.*

must be so good with food, to which I respond, "Don't let someone's appearance fool you." There are many thin people with terrible diets, and overweight people who eat well. You never know what someone's relationship to food is, until they tell you.

June 19, 2017
My clients at the gym tell me about their food struggles and say, "Oh well, you have such good food control," etc. And I say, "No. I know what it's

like to be addicted to food." In my first year at Waterloo University, there were two Tim Horton's coffee shops on campus. Tim's had their cookies on sale by the half-dozen, promoting them because they were new back then. I've always liked cookies and these cookies looked amazing – soft, chewy, chocolate. I thought I would just try some.

Trying some eventually turned into 30 days with six Tim's cookies per day. At the end of the month I had ballooned out and felt like garbage – tired, mind fog and grumpy. Then with cookie in hand I looked down and thought, oh my God! It's the cookies. I need to stop. Not to mention that this was becoming an expensive habit not easily managed during student life.

Looking back, I realize this is also where I developed my secret eating pattern, which is a form of disordered eating. Anyway, I had intense cravings and constantly went back and forth in my head saying, "Oh well, I can just have it once in a while. I'm ok." Ultimately, I had to change the routes I walked around school completely, and I told a friend about the cookies for some moral support. To this day I hesitate buying Tim's cookies.

Going back to disordered eating for a moment, disordered eating means much more than anorexia and bulimia. While teaching the canfitpro™ course, Healthy Eating and Weight Loss Coach, I learned that disordered eating comes in many forms. For example, distracted eating while driving or watching

TV, or the over-exercisers who eat something they feel guilty about and try to work it off at the gym. Others eat quickly, not taking the time to taste and enjoy the food, or they use food as comfort. These examples may seem benign, but when done frequently, they cause problems, such as overeating, or choosing the wrong foods because you're in a hurry. It even extends to hurting yourself or getting sick from an overuse injury at the gym, or a suppressed immune system from all the cortisol in your system from over exercising.

I know I associate food with tradition, but I had no idea that it also plays a factor in my happiness. I hate to admit it, but it became glaringly obvious when I went on a road trip this past year prior to my May 2017 competition. For as long as I can remember, on family trips we always made stops at rest stations and it was a special occasion because I got to choose any place I wanted to stop to eat on these trips. I could even choose places with fast food, which I almost never got otherwise.

As an adult I realized it is now engrained in me that *road trip* means *junk food*. On this particular road trip, while in training for my first show, I had to pack all my food and stick to it while others had Taco Bell and Michigan Coneys. On the trip I was having fun, but it wasn't the usual excitement. It was as if my fun had been dampened with the change of food.

Another big lesson was that no matter how much you plan and prepare for show day, you must be prepared for unexpected things to happen and be able to roll with whatever comes. This is much easier said than done. Be warned, anything can come up. Other competitors gave me some examples. One bikini competitor had a seizure induced by a head injury she sustained from a car accident, months before. She had lingering concussion symptoms one week before the show, and she still competed!

My own experiences included not being able to move my back for a week and a half before the first show and the mad dash it was to fit in all the chiropractic and massage treatments I could. Before the second show I got a cold that lasted up until a week and a half before the competition. Also, my stand-in coach texted me on the Wednesday, with only three sleeps until show day, to tell me she was sick. At first I panicked thinking, OMG, I don't know how to do makeup and I don't want to be alone backstage. It wasn't good. My other friend who was coming to the show volunteered to step in if needed. Thank goodness. Always have a contingency plan.

> *Be cautious of which show you decide to do. If it is your first show, have as many people there as possible to cheer you on.*

Shows are being held all over Ontario in most months of the year. Be cautious of which show you decide to do. If it is your first show, I recommend having as many people there as possible to cheer you on. That means the date of the show will matter, not only for the holidays that you may miss in between, but also because some shows fall on long weekends or holidays. For example, the KWOSHOW that I did this year was on Thanksgiving weekend. Several people who enjoy the shows wanted to go but already had family plans. As mentioned before, there is never a good time for everyone, but planning makes it the best it can be.

Conclusion

"The 3 C's in life: Choice, Chance, Change. You must make the Choice, to take the Chance, if you want anything in life to Change."

– curiano.com

I'm so thankful for this journey. My New Year resolutions are few and far between, so making one in 2015 I knew I had to fulfill it somehow. The support in achieving my goal has been amazing. The best part about the shows for me is that I walked away knowing I accomplished something tough, really tough, and I exceeded my expectations of myself. I never knew I could be so strong, physically and mentally. Having said that, two shows in one year is a lot, especially for a newbie. So, if you win, be ready for it!

The fitness competition industry was another world to me, with new rules and customs to follow. I used to look at the women who did them and think I'd never be able to do that. Yet here I am with two shows under my belt. I am in awe of what the body can do and how it withstands all the stress we inflict. I'm glad I chose to avoid the usual supplements because I don't have to worry about any potential health consequences later on. Competing in a show is achieving a big goal. All your hard work – literally blood, sweat and tears – has gone into it, but it is only one day. The months of preparation and the aftermath are what you have to live.

Be safe. Make sure you pick the right team to back you up, and have supporters to help you along the way. Once you get the competition bug, you'll be hooked. My friends are already taking bets on whether or not I will do a third show. For now, I'm focusing on what fitness means to me, rather than an ideal set by someone else.

Fitness to me is more than just the physical. It is mental wellbeing, physical strength and endurance, as well as overall health. I can't see fitness without health since you need one to truly have the other. In order for me to achieve this, I need more balance when it comes to career, gym and relaxation so this is what I'm working toward now.

> *Fitness is more than just the physical – it is physical strength and endurance, but also mental well being and overall health.*

Choosing to step into the fitness world is truly a mental, emotional and physical ride! Keep your health in mind and push your body to its natural limits.

"Note to self: you gotta do this for you. This is for you. This isn't about anybody. Live for you. Honor you. Never lose sight of that."

– theberry.com

References

*(Canadian Fitness Professionals, Inc.)

Nana by Trey Songz.
https://www.youtube.com/watch?v=v0Gu_Yh_keE)

NaturopathicallyFit Channel.
https://www.youtube.com/channel/UCKaAUhSdM-htuS9jz9yUWIQ

Bresan, Paola and Kramer, Peter. "Bread and Other Edible Agents of Mental Disease," Frontiers in Human Neuroscience. March 2016.

Appendix: Quick Reference for a Full Body Stretch

Stretch, Stretch and Stretch again! I'm a huge advocate for stretching. It is one of the most under-used healing techniques and is one of the easiest because it doesn't cost a thing and you can do it anywhere. If you don't want to take the time post-workout to do it, take breaks at work to fit it in, do it while watching TV, or before going to bed. Incorporate deep breathing, dim the lights and you will be ready for bed!

Some people are in the stretch-before-working-out camp. Only use this method after a five- to ten-minute warm-up and have it be more dynamic. That means, taking your body through the movements and ranges of motion that you are working on that day. For example, if you are working on your back, do some side bends, then forward flexion by slowly reaching for your toes and rolling up slowly. Then reach your arms out in front of you and pull them back, mimicking a rowing motion.

Your workout intensity level dictates how much stretching you need to do. Take more time to stretch a problem area, if you have one. When preparing for a show, dynamic stretching is not enough. You also need to stretch post-workout. This stretching is more static, meaning you hold the pose and allow the muscle to lengthen. Use caution when stretching. **It's not good to bounce in a static stretch or to feel any pain.** The discomfort of a stretch should never be more than two on a pain scale from zero to ten, with 10 being painful and 0 representing no pain. If you feel anything more than that, ease back out of the stretch until it is comfortable again.

Even if you are doing the split training method – working two or three muscle groups per session, I still highly recommend doing a full body stretch at the end of every workout. Even on an arms and shoulders day, you still use your legs for the cardio, and on a back and chest day, you still use your arms for pushing and pulling. Either way you look at it, you use your whole body at some point, and stretching daily gives attention to any muscles that are still tense or didn't get enough stretching the previous day.

Before the injury I got a week and a half previous to my show, I used to stretch 10 minutes per session, now I do a full body stretch for about 15 minutes allowing a little extra in case a certain area needs more stretching. **Hold each stretch for at least 45 seconds.** I recommend timing yourself because people tend to count quickly to get stretching over with. Keep in mind it is going to help ease muscle recovery, loosen tense muscles and minimize next day soreness.

Until I got serious about doing a competition, I had no idea about the fitness competition world. With my own experience and hearing many stories from other competitors, I've learned A LOT! I hope that you can learn from my mistakes and that your competition journey is happy, healthy and strong.

Seated Latissimus Dorsi (large back muscle) Stretch

Start:

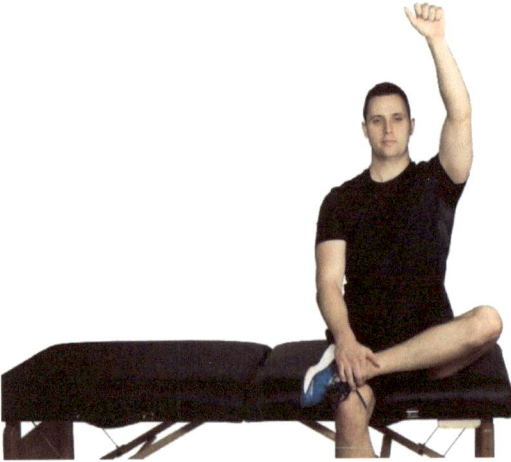

End:

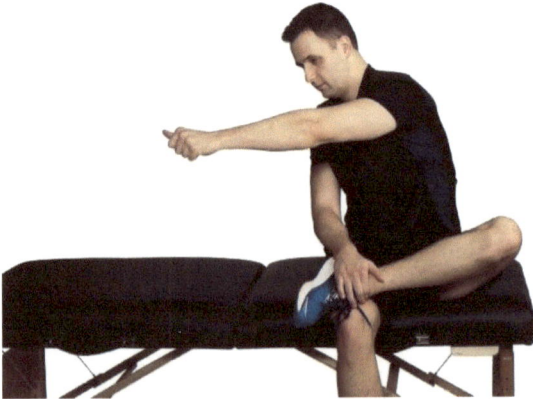

Gastrocnemius (calf) Stretch

The back leg is the one getting the stretch. Drive your heel into the floor, keeping the leg straight. To stretch the Soleus muscle (the calf muscle under the Gastrocnemius), bend the back knee while continuing to keep your heel to the floor.

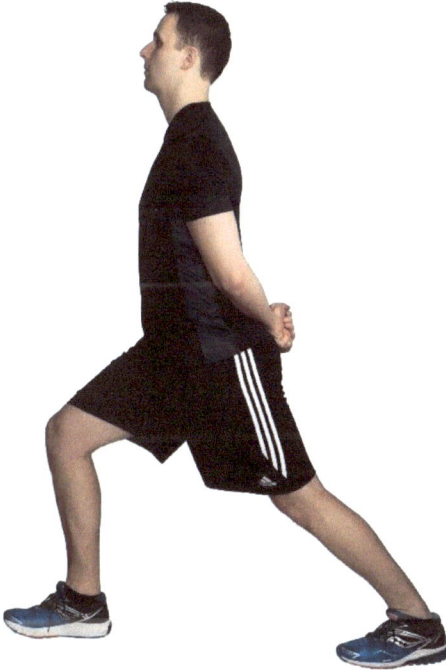

Pectoralis Major (Chest) Stretch

Have your legs in a lunge position to help with balance. Ensure your arm is at 90 degrees, lean into the wall to feel more of a stretch.

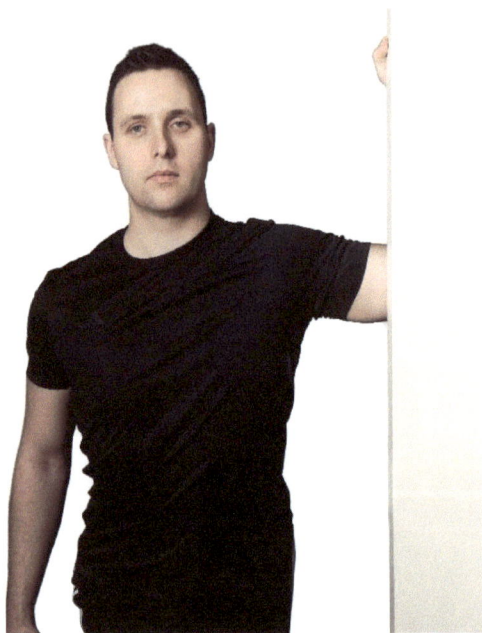

Quadriceps (front of thigh) Stretch

Aim to keep the thighs parallel. When the quads are very tight, people tend to have their knee pointing to the outside rather than down.

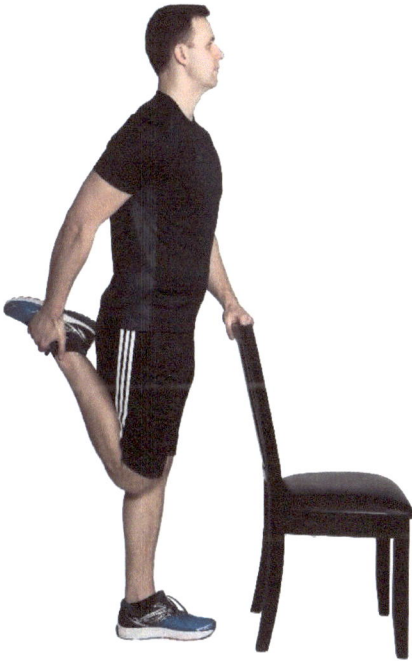

Hamstrings (back of thigh) Stretch

This stretch can be done seated, as seen here, or standing and reaching down to the toes as far as you can. The key here is to stretch toward your toes WITHOUT bouncing. Bouncing can lead to muscle strain and even tear. Go slowly and stop where you feel a good stretch with no pain.

Hip Flexor (deep muscle, front of thigh) Stretch

Also called the runner's stretch. Lean into the stretch with your hips while keeping your posture nice and tall. If this bothers your knee, you can place a towel just below the kneecap to reduce the pressure.

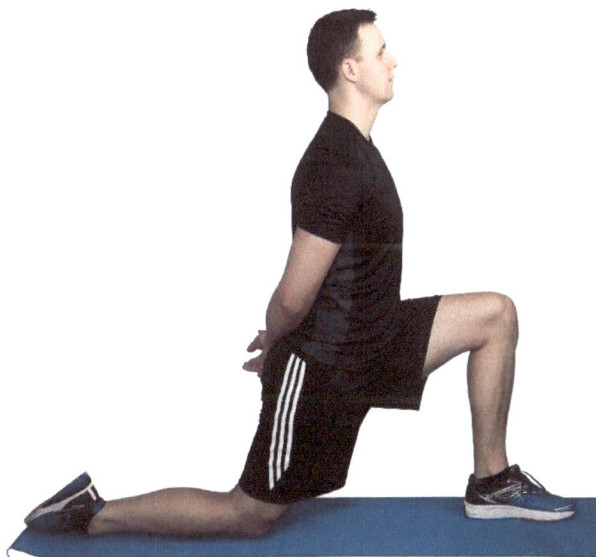

Piriformis (glutes) Stretch

Aim to keep your back in neutral spine and bend at the hips. Only lean forward as far as you can without rounding the back.

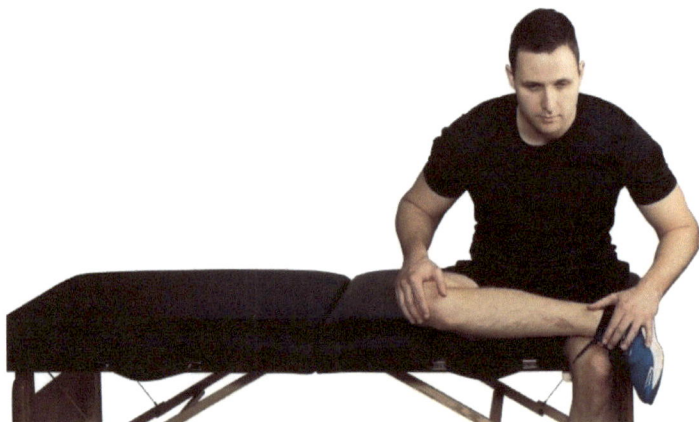

Biceps (front of upper arm) Stretch

The bicep muscle's primary action is to supinate the hand (to bring the hand palm up, as if carrying a bowl of soup) so you need to ensure that you are stretching with your arm straight, and the thumb is in contact with the surface you are using to stretch.

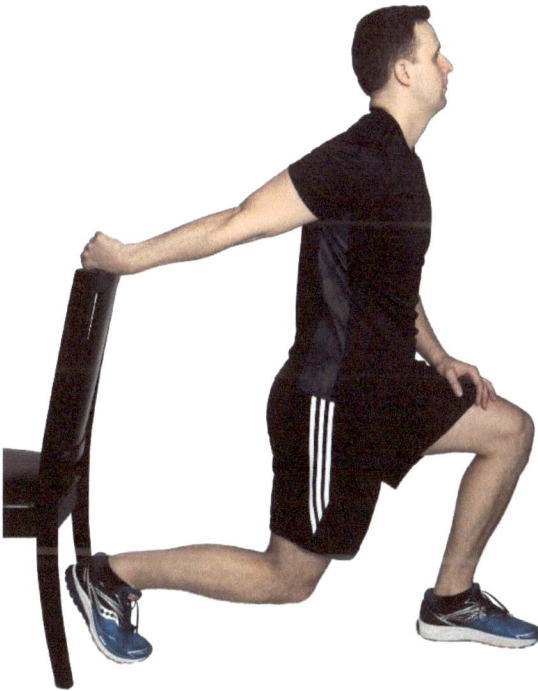

Dr. Katelyn Butler-Birmingham

Triceps (back of upper arm) Stretch

Use the hand pushing down on the opposite elbow to stretch a little further – the fingertips of the stretching arm will slide down the upper back.

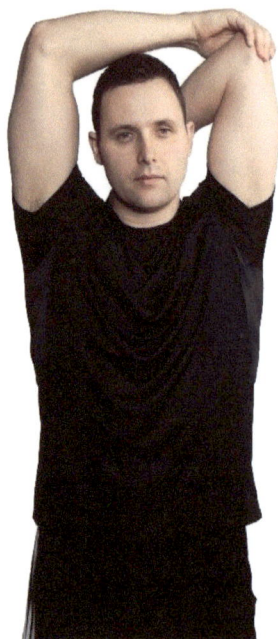

Photo Credits:
   Chris Smith, Registered Massage Therapy
   Kamini Le Capelain of Silent Poetry

About the Author

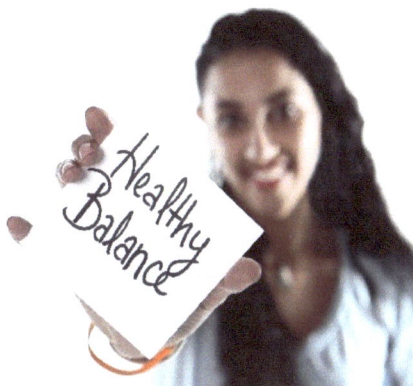

Dr. Katelyn Butler-Birmingham had an early introduction to Naturopathic Medicine from her Mom, and found that the treatments and time spent with the Naturopathic Doctor created a safe, open and healing experience unlike any other.

She studied Kinesiology Pre-Health with Co-op option at the University of Waterloo. Dr. K wanted to incorporate her love of science, sport and health, so went on to study Naturopathic Medicine at the Canadian College of Naturopathic Medicine. She was on the Sports Medicine shift.

To explore a new challenge, she ventured into the fitness competition world – a world where "Natural" means many things, including using fat burners, caffeine pills, diuretics and even steroids to get results. If you want to navigate the competition scene

Dr. Katelyn Butler-Birmingham

and see what your body really can do Naturally, this book is for you!

www.naturopathicallyfit.com

Facebook: Dr. Katelyn Butler-Birmingham, BSc Kin, ND

Twitter @KTBB_ND

Instagram @naturopathicallyfit

www.ingramcontent.com/pod-product-compliance
Lightning Source LLC
Chambersburg PA
CBHW040131270326
41929CB00001B/2